The Five Senses:

A Sensible Guide to Sensory Loss

Kathy N. Johnson, PhD, CMC

James H. Johnson, PhD

Lily Sarafan, MS

All Rights Reserved. No part of this book may be used or reproduced in any matter without the written permission of the Publisher. Printed in the United States of America. For information address Home Care Press, 148 Hawthorne Avenue, Palo Alto, CA 94301.

ISBN 978-0-9857236-0-6

OTHER BOOKS BY THE AUTHORS

Happy to 102: The Best Kept Secrets to a Long and Happy Life

The Handbook of Live-in Care: A Guide for Caregivers

From Hospital to Home Care: A Step by Step Guide to Providing Care to Patients Post Hospitalization

Comfort Foods Cookbook: A Healthy Twist on Classic Favorites.

ACKNOWLEDGMENTS

This book is dedicated to all those who embrace a positive view of aging, particularly the family and professional caregivers who brighten the lives of older adults on a daily basis.

TABLE OF CONTENTS

TABLE OF CONTENTS

INTRODUCTION

Most of us are born with five functioning senses and ways of experiencing the world around us. These senses include hearing, vision, touch, smell and taste. Our senses may change over our lifespans for various reasons. As your eyes develop, for instance, you may experience vision difficulties such as astigmatism or near-sightedness because the lens of your eye isn't curved correctly. Being exposed to loud noises can cause damage to your ears that results in hearing impairment. Illness or injury may affect your sense of touch. And some medications, such as certain types of chemotherapy given to cancer patients, can temporarily or permanently impair your ability to taste or smell.

Old age brings predictable changes to our senses, often making them less sharp and less able to accurately supply our brain with information about what is going on around us. If you are caring for an older adult, you need to be aware of how the senses may change with age. This is important for several reasons.

First, behavior caused by hearing loss may be incorrectly attributed to disease. People who do not hear well may answer questions inappropriately or fail to follow simple conversations. Because this kind of "confusion", which is also typical of the early stages of dementia, it is important to rule out hearing loss before making a diagnosis of Alzheimer's disease or some other dementia.

Another reason you need to be aware of sensory change is that loss of smell and/or taste may affect your loved one's appetite. If the older adult you are caring for begins refusing favorite foods, it is possible that the once-loved foods no longer taste good. They may be too bland, or they may simply have a different taste than he or she is used to. As your loved one's sense of taste changes, you will have to experiment to find new favorite foods.

Finally, a decline in vision or touch can present a safety risk for older adults. If the person you are caring for can no longer see well, he or she may become vulnerable to tripping and falling, especially in unfamiliar environments. Seniors with declining visual acuity may also accidentally leave appliances running if they can no longer see the off/on switch.

If your loved one's sense of touch has been damaged by a stroke or other medical condition, such as diabetic neuropathy, he may not be able to feel his foot making contact with the ground. With little or no sense of touch to guide him, he may accidentally place his weight on the side of his foot and stumble, or he might tangle his feet, resulting in a fall.

A final reason to be aware of changes in the five senses that may occur with old age is that your loved one may be reluctant to admit that her senses are not as sharp as they once were. She may be too proud to admit she needs help now, or she may fear losing her independence and being placed in a nursing facility.

If you recognize that a certain amount of sensory loss is a normal part of aging, you can be on the lookout for warning signs and help your loved one identify ways to cope before these deficits become dangerous.

An Overview of the Five Senses

This book is set up in five sections, each devoted to a different sense. The first chapter in each section will explain how each sense receives and processes input from the environment. This is meant to provide you with a working knowledge of the sense and familiarize you with terms that you may hear associated with it. The second chapter will address some of the common sensory problems we experience as we age. Understanding the various age-related sensory problems and dysfunctions will make you more attuned to spotting problems earlier in a loved one. Finally, the third chapter will provide tips for helping your loved one compensate for sensory deficits by making some simple lifestyle changes, using assistive equipment, or providing additional support in the form of a professional caregiver from a home care agency such as Home Care Assistance, to help with tasks such as writing letters or completing household chores.

With well-planned assistance and your empathetic understanding, your loved one can remain in his or her home and maintain a sense of independence in spite of the sensory deficits that often accompany advanced age.

What is Home Care?

Throughout this book, we mention home care and how professional caregivers can help maintain your loved one's independence and enhance his or her quality of life. This might be a good place to delve a little deeper into what exactly home care is. There are two types of home care: medical and non-medical.

Medical home care describes services delivered by nurses and licensed physical, occupational and speech therapists. Recipients must be homebound and have a skilled medical need, such as wound care or intravenous antibiotics. Medical home care is intermittent, meaning that the caregivers make visits a few times per week, typically on a short-term, temporary basis.

When we discuss home care in this book, we are most often referring to non-medical care. Non-medical home care describes a service where another person, usually a family member, friend, or paid caregiver, provides a senior assistance with activities of daily living, such as dressing and bathing and with household tasks such as preparing meals or running errands.

The need for non-medical home care has skyrocketed since 1995. This was the first year records showed more people dying from chronic conditions than from acute diseases. With acute illnesses claiming fewer lives, life expectancy has increased sharply. Most seniors today can expect to live the majority of their lives, at home, in good health. While aging adults are living longer and more productive lives than ever, the onset of chronic health conditions such as heart disease, kidney failure, dementia, or sensory losses can make remaining in the comfort of home a challenge.

When these conditions occur, aging adults may be unable to continue living in their own home without assistance. In the past, this meant moving in with a family member or being transferred to an assisted living facility or nursing home—in spite of the fact that numerous aging surveys have found that a staggering 90% of seniors have an expressed wish to continue living in their own homes and "age in place."

Non-medical home care can make that wish a reality by providing personalized assistance tailored to keep the senior safe and comfortable in a non-institutional setting.

Some of the services provided by non-medical caregivers include help with eating, bathing, toileting, managing incontinence, remaining as mobile as possible, performing light housekeeping duties, and providing or arranging transportation. Non-medical caregivers can also provide medication reminders.

Caregivers can be hired on an as-needed basis. Some families hire caregivers for just a few hours each week so that the family member providing care can take a much-deserved break, referred to as respite care. Other families may require caregivers for several hours each day or around-the-clock. It is not at all unusual for a senior whose health is in decline to require a live-in caregiver.

Typically, when you call a home care agency like Home Care Assistance, they will meet with you and your loved one to find out exactly what services you need and to establish a unique, personalized care plan. They will then assign a caregiver and arrange an introductory meeting to ensure that the caregiver and your loved one are a good match.

When Is It Time for Non-Medical Home Care?

Many senior citizens and their families find the decision making process around the ideal time to bring on a caregiver daunting. The best advice we can offer is to hire one sooner rather than later. This gives your loved one a chance to develop a strong rapport with the caregiver so that he or she will be more accepting of the caregiver's assistance as care needs increase. Many people wait until a crisis has occurred, for example, a fall or unexpected hospitalization, to begin looking for assistance from a home care agency. It's important to be proactive in researching care options and developing a relationship with a care agency before a crisis occurs.

There are also a few signs to watch for that will alert you to the fact that your loved one needs extra help in the home, including:

- **Messy home.** Some people are simply neater than others, but if you notice an unusual amount of clutter, piled up garbage, or stacks of undone dishes, it may be time to think about getting your loved one extra help.

- **Strange odors.** Odd smells in the house may indicate spoiled food, an inability to care for pets, or a problem with incontinence. A professional caregiver can help with all of these problems.

- **Poor hygiene.** This can include unwashed or messy hair, unwashed clothing, body odor, or wearing clothes that are unsuitable to the occasion or the weather. For example, if your loved one chooses to wear shorts to run errands in a snowstorm, he or she may be suffering from cognitive problems or a medical condition that keeps him or her from noticing dangerously cold temperatures.

- **Driving problems.** Problems with driving can include minor accidents, unexplained scratches or dents on the car, or more than one ticket issued in a three month time period. Take notice when you ride with your loved one. If he or she does not pay attention to the road, ignores or fails to see traffic signals, or weaves between lanes, it's probably time to find someone else to do the driving and errand-running.

- **Dramatic weight loss or gain.** A weight change of more than 10% can signal that your loved one is making poor nutritional decisions or is simply physically unable to prepare healthy meals. It could also signify depression, which should be addressed immediately.

- **Isolation.** Withdrawing from friends and family can be a sign of sensory deficits like hearing problems, or it might indicate a problem with cognition or mental health. An in-home caregiver can provide not only physical services, but also the socialization your loved one needs.

Caregiver Options

It is natural to want to provide care to your loved one by yourself. After all, who knows your mother or father better than you do? However, acting as the sole caregiver to your loved one can take a toll on your well-being. In fact, some studies suggest that the rate of depression among family caregivers is as high as 70%. Also, if you are not trained to provide care to a dependent senior, you could accidentally injure yourself or your loved one. Finally, many family members report a sense of loss at feeling that the special familial or romantic relationship they held with their loved one has been compromised because of the care provider/care recipient dynamic; for example, it is quite common for the adult child of a parent who needs care to feel that bringing on additional support allows them to regain at least some component of that special child/parent relationship they thought was lost.

Another option is hiring a caregiver privately. While this option has worked for families, there are also certain risks and complications. Suppose, for instance, that the caregiver you hire turns out to be unreliable or unprofessional and simply fails to show up on some days. While an agency has an on-call scheduler to quickly adapt to these instances and provide alternate care so your loved is never left alone, this burden falls onto your shoulders if you do not have the support of an agency. As an employer, it is also up to you to be aware of tax, workmen's compensation, and employment laws.

A third option is to hire a non-medical home care agency. Hiring a high-caliber agency can remove a tremendous amount of the caregiving burden from your shoulders. Since the agency employs the caregivers, you won't need to worry about issues like withholding taxes or paying unemployment if you have to dismiss a caregiver.

Additionally, a good agency will make every effort to match your loved one with a compatible caregiver. The agency will also make sure that your loved one's needs are met even if the regularly scheduled caregiver is ill or unavailable.

Who Pays?

Non-medical home care is not covered by Medicare or by health insurance. It is covered by many long-term care insurance plans, however.

The other alternative is for your loved one to pay for the care privately, an option most families end up using. Although the costs may seem steep at first glance, they are generally less than the costs of having your loved one cared for in a nursing home or an assisted living facility. It is also worth the extra money to help your loved one remain in his or her home for life.

If your loved one does not have the resources to pay for private care, you might consider getting several family members to agree to pay a small percentage of the cost of home care each month; this is a nice approach for many families in order to distribute the costs among siblings and other relatives paying for the care.

The Bottom Line

If your loved one is like 89% of the senior population, he or she will prefer to age in his or her own home. A good non-medical home care agency can fulfill that desire by providing services that allow your loved one to get all of the care he or she needs without the trauma that often comes with leaving familiar surroundings and moving to a facility.

HEARING

CHAPTER 1.1: HOW OUR EARS WORK

Even before birth, our sense of hearing is an integral component of how we interact with the world. Studies suggest that a fetus's hearing develops at about sixteen weeks of age, at the same time the small bones in the middle ear are formed. A fetus who hears the same music repeatedly while in the womb will show signs of recognizing the familiar tune after he or she is born.

Our ears are constructed so they can distinguish a loved one's whisper that signals comfort from a sharp cry that signals danger. Working in conjunction with our brains, our ears can pick up on subtle innuendos such as the subtle annoyance in the voice of a spouse or the sadness in the voice of a friend who is trying to act cheerful.

How Sound Travels

The sense of hearing is actually based on vibrations and the physical movements of particles through the air.

The pitch of a sound—that is, whether we consider a sound to be high or low—has to do with the frequency of the sound waves coming at us. High-frequency sound waves result in a high pitch, while low-frequency sound waves result in a lower pitch.

Some sound waves vibrate so quickly and frequently that the human ear cannot even register them, although many animals are able to hear these high pitches. Think about a dog whistle; you cannot hear the sound it makes, but whenever you blow it, your furry friend comes running.

The other way that sounds differ is in terms of loudness. How loud a sound is depends upon the level of pressure or the amount of force exerted on the vibrating particles. When you yell, for instance, remember how your chest and throat sometimes ache from exerting so much pressure on the air around you. This does not happen when you speak in a soft monotone, because you are exercising less pressure.

The Structure of the Ears

How do our ears capture these vibrations and turn them into meaningful pieces of information? To understand this process, you must first understand the structure of the ear itself, which is comprised of three parts: the external ear, the middle ear and the inner ear.

The External Ear

The external ear is composed of an oval-shaped piece of cartilage called the pinna. The pinna's job is to collect vibrations or sounds. Due to the shape and position of our pinna, humans are better able to collect sounds that are in front of them. Cats, dogs, and other animals can actually swivel their pinna so they can collect vibrations from any direction. For instance, the next time you approach your cat from behind and make an unexpected noise, watch how his ears swivel to catch the sound.

Once the pinna has captured the vibration or sound, it passes the vibration along to the eardrum or the tympanic membrane, another feature of the external ear. The eardrum is about an inch long and less than a quarter of an inch in diameter. It is made up of thin, taut layers of skin, much like the surface of a drum. When the eardrum receives vibrations from the pinna, it immediately passes them on to the middle ear.

The Middle Ear

The middle ear is an air-filled space that contains structures called ossicles to help amplify sound. It also contains three of the smallest bones in the human body—the malleus, the stapes, and the incus—all of which play a significant role in passing sound vibrations to the inner ear.

The middle ear is connected to the back of the throat by the Eustachian tube. This tube helps ensure that the pressure in the middle ear and the air pressure are roughly equivalent. As children, many people experience colds and infections that block the Eustachian tubes. These illnesses are often the cause of earaches. They can also lead to temporary hearing loss, though hearing usually returns to normal once the infection is gone.

The Inner Ear

The inner ear is made up of two main structures: the cochlea, which controls our ability to hear, and the vestibule, which controls our balance. Problems with the vestibule cause some people with inner ear infections to feel dizzy or even to fall.

The cochlea is a small part of the ear. Shaped much like a snail, it is embedded in protective bone and filled with fluid. The cochlea also contains the organ of Corti, which is lined with sensitive hair cells. These cells detect sound waves and transform them into electrical impulses.

The electrical signals make their way up the auditory nerve to the auditory cortex of the brain. The brain translates the complex electronic code into meaningful and recognizable sounds, like speech, laughter, or a loud clap of thunder.

As you can see, processing sound requires several different structures in the ear and the brain to work closely with each other. If any of those structures become damaged or stop functioning properly, our sense of hearing suffers.

It is little wonder that hearing loss is a common problem among older adults. The next chapter examines the causes and symptoms of adult hearing loss.

CHAPTER 1.2: COMMON HEARING PROBLEMS

The Mayo Clinic estimates that one in three people in the United States between the ages of 65 and 75 and more than half of all people older than 75 suffer from some type of hearing loss. According to the Canadian Hard of Hearing Association, more than 40% of Canadians over the age of 65 experience some type of hearing loss. There are many different reasons why our sense of hearing may become impaired as we age.

Presbycusis

Presbycusis is an umbrella term that refers to the slow, irreversible hearing loss that many people suffer as they grow older. Scientists say that the most likely culprit is the decline of the tiny hair cells in the organ of Corti in the inner ear. With these cells dead or damaged, electrical impulses have a much harder time reaching the auditory cortex where sounds can be processed and referred to other areas of the brain for appropriate responses.

Researchers are unsure why these tiny hair cells suffer damage as we age. It may be because, like the hair on our heads, the hairs in the organ of Corti naturally age and become thin and brittle over the years.

Presbycusis has also been linked to various risk factors including a family history of hearing loss, repeated exposure to loud noises and cigarette smoking.

Ear Wax (Cerumen)

Ear wax, or cerumen, is a substance secreted close to the eardrum in the external ear. Its function is to clean and lubricate the ear and to protect the sensitive structures of the middle ear and the inner ear from infection. Ear wax is usually self-cleaning. Once it has served its purpose, it will dry up and be expelled from the outer ear in small flakes that are almost invisible to the naked eye.

Ironically, hearing loss due to ear wax blockage usually does not become a problem unless a person uses a cotton-tipped stick or a similar object to try to remove the ear wax. Instead of removing it, they usually only succeed in pushing dry wax deeper into the ear where it becomes stuck and impairs hearing.

Luckily, cerumen blocks do not cause permanent harm. They usually clear themselves if you put a few drops of mineral oil or baby oil into the ear for a little extra lubrication. More serious impactions can be irrigated by a doctor or caregiver acting under the doctor's instructions.

Ototoxic Medications

Ototoxics are medicines known to result in either temporary or permanent hearing loss. Researchers have identified over 200 types of ototoxic medications. Most are used to treat severe, antibiotic-resistant infections, heart disease, or cancer. Before your loved one starts a new medication, ask the doctor about side effects including hearing loss. Ask the doctor what steps he or she will recommend if your loved one does experience hearing loss while taking the medication. Sometimes lowering the dose or switching to a different medicine can relieve this problem.

Acoustic Neuroma

An acoustic neuroma is a slow-growing, non-cancerous tumor that attaches itself to the vestibular cochlear nerve in the inner ear. The main symptom of acoustic neuroma is slow, progressive hearing loss that occurs in just one ear. Treatment depends on the size of the tumor and on the amount of distress it causes the afflicted person. The most common treatment options include medication and surgery, though sometimes a physician may recommend "watchful waiting", or observation.

Meniere's Disease

Meniere's disease is a distressing condition that results in balance and hearing problems. Victims may experience dizziness, nausea and vomiting, or ringing and significant hearing loss in one ear. Doctors do not fully understand Meniere's disease, but they suspect it has something to do with an increase of pressure within the inner ear.

Conductive Hearing Loss

Conductive hearing loss is typically seen in younger patients, though it can affect people of all ages. Conductive hearing loss occurs when sound is not properly conducted through the ear drum or the middle ear. The victim usually complains of hearing loss in one ear as well as a feeling of the ear being "plugged up."

Several problems can cause conductive hearing loss including a punctured eardrum, fluid build-up in the middle ear, or even a genetic malformation. The problem can usually be resolved by corrective surgery.

Symptoms of Hearing Loss

In some cases, your loved one may simply tell you that he or she is having trouble understanding speech or hearing different types of sounds. In other cases, though, they may be embarrassed by his or her hearing loss and try to hide it from you.

If you watch your loved one's behavior, you will probably see several symptoms and signs that tip you off about a possible hearing problem. Examples include:

- Difficulty understanding certain words
- Giving answers that don't make sense in the context of the question
- Frequently asking people to repeat themselves
- Playing the television, CD player, or radio so loudly that it becomes a nuisance to neighbors
- Withdrawing from conversation
- Avoiding certain social situations
- Not hearing certain sounds like a doorbell or a ringing telephone

Getting Help

Taken together, these signs point to a hearing problem, but individually, they could also be caused by other factors. A person who cannot answer a question appropriately, for instance, might be suffering from dementia, and withdrawing from social situations can be a sign of depression. That is why you should first consult your loved one's general practitioner. He or she can perform a full medical checkup.

If your loved one's doctor finds that hearing loss is a problem, he or she will probably refer you to an ear, nose, and throat specialist (ENT) or to an audiologist for additional testing and possibly a hearing aid.

The next chapter will describe the ways that you as a caregiver can help your hearing-impaired loved one continue to lead a full and enjoyable life.

CHAPTER 1.3: COMPENSATING FOR HEARING PROBLEMS

If your loved one suffers from hearing loss, there are several ways that you can help him or her compensate and continue to function as normally as possible. The treatment of hearing loss depends upon the cause, but don't be surprised if your loved one's GP, ENT, or audiologist recommends a hearing aid.

Hearing Aids

Hearing aids are small, unobtrusive devices that rest on, or just inside, the external ear. They process and amplify sounds as they pass to the middle ear and the inner ear. A hearing aid consists of at least four distinct components:

1. The microphone, much like the pinna, detects and collects sounds.
2. The amplifier increases the volume of certain sounds.
3. The speaker then sends those amplified sounds into the ear where they can be processed and transmitted to the brain.
4. A small battery acts as the power source.

There are two basic kinds of hearing aids available on the market. The older is the analog, which turns sounds into amplified electronic signals. The newer model of hearing aid, the digital hearing aid, converts symbols into binary numbers. These numbers can actually help distinguish important sounds, like your spouse asking you a question, from unimportant sounds, like a bird chirping outside your window.

Reluctant Consumers

A 2010 study published in the journal Gerontology found that hearing aids were effective in helping people with mild to moderate hearing loss, especially if they are professionally fitted and calibrated. Unfortunately, the study also found that only about 20% of Americans, who could benefit from hearing aids, actually wore them. The Social and Aboriginal Statistics Division in Canada reported that 19% of Canadians with hearing loss used hearing aids or other assistive devices.

Two of the most common reasons seniors, who are hard of hearing, don't wear hearing aids are embarrassment and cost. It may help your loved one to go to a hearing clinic and see just how small today's hearing aids really are. It's unlikely that a casual acquaintance would even notice the hearing aid. There's even a joke making the rounds about an audiologist who fitted his patient with a hearing aid and asked him to come back in a week to see how things were going. The older man returned a week later with a twinkle in his eye and said that he was enjoying being able to hear clearly for the first time in a decade.

"That's great!" the audiologist said. "What does your family think?"

"Oh, they don't know I have it," said the man, "but I've changed my will four times since last Monday."

Cost is also a factor that prevents some seniors from purchasing hearing aids. If your loved one is afraid he or she can't afford the device, take some time to shop around at various hearing clinics and locate the most reasonable prices. When you visit the clinics, you might also ask if there are any city, county, or state funds available to help seniors finance the purchase of hearing aids.

Finally, while it is probably not the best idea to buy the cheapest hearing aids on the market, you probably don't need to buy the most expensive pair either. Shoot for a mid-range device, and you'll likely strike the optimal balance between cost and quality.

Hearing Aid Tips:

As soon as your loved one gets his or her hearing aid, take some time to read through the instructions, especially the parts having to do with maintenance. Make sure to keep the device clean of ear wax and to check the batteries on a regular basis. Read the following tips to get started:

- If your loved one doesn't like the way the hearing aid feels, encourage him or her to wear it for a few hours every day. The longer they wear it, the sooner he or she will get used to it.

- If your loved one has a digital hearing aid, it will adjust itself automatically to different levels of sound. Your loved one should not have to make any manual adjustments.

- Make sure you always keep a supply of batteries on hand.

- Pick a place to store the hearing aid. Because hearing aids are so small, they can be easily lost or thrown away. Some people wrap them in a tissue to keep them safe and then accidentally put the tissue in the waste basket. Pick a memorable location like a jewelry box or a brightly colored tin container and get into the habit of placing the hearing aid there whenever it is not in use.

Other Devices

If your loved one finds the hearing aid helpful, there are other types of assistive technology he or she might also find useful.

A telephone amplifying device, for instance, contains a special receiver that amplifies the voice of the person to whom you are speaking.

If she still enjoys watching television, ask the hearing clinic about an amplifying head phone device so she can watch television without disturbing neighbors or other people in the house. In some places, you may also be able to arrange closed captioning for the majority of programs through your cable company.

Finally, if your loved one has trouble hearing the high frequencies of the telephone and the doorbell, try purchasing a device that flashes colored lights or vibrates in your loved one's pocket to alert him or her of a visitor or a phone call.

Cochlear Implants

Used mainly in cases of profound hearing loss, which involves damage to the inner ear, the cochlear implant is a small, electronic device that is surgically placed just under the skin behind the ear. Basically, the device bypasses the inner ear and sends messages directly to the brain for processing.

Final Tips to Help Your Loved One Compensate for Hearing Loss

- When you speak to your loved one, either face him or her head on or, if hearing is better in one ear than in the other, speak directly into their good ear.
- Talk clearly, at a normal speed.

- Do not yell or shout. Yelling makes you sound angry, even if that is not your intent.

- Do not cover your mouth as you talk. Some people who have suffered slow hearing loss over a long period of time have taught themselves to read lips.

- Use facial expressions and gestures, as well as words, to communicate.

- Do not talk about the person who has a hearing problem. Talk to him or her. If you need to share private information with a third party, beckon that person outside the room.

- Lowering the pitch of your voice may make it easier for your loved one to hear you.

- Reduce background noise before starting a conversation with your loved one.

- Just because your loved one nods, don't assume he or she understands. Ask your loved one to repeat the message back to you.

- Don't become tired or frustrated with your loved one. Instead, stay calm and work with them to figure out the best ways to communicate.

HOW HOME CARE CAN HELP

1. Checking batteries and keep hearing aids clean. This is especially important if your loved one has cognitive problems like Alzheimer's disease or if he or she has other sensory deficiencies that make handling the small hearing aids difficult.

2. Help with socialization. Many people with hearing loss withdraw from social situations because they are embarrassed if they don't understand what is said to them or if they have to ask someone to repeat themselves. A caregiver can quickly learn the best ways to communicate with your loved one and the two of them should be able to have at least some enjoyable interaction each day.

3. Attending medical appointments. If your loved one doesn't hear well, he or she may not understand everything the doctor says. If you can't go to appointments with loved ones on your own, ask the caregiver to go and take careful notes which you can review later.

4. Teaching assistive equipment use. A caregiver can teach your loved one how to use technology like a telecommunications device for the deaf (TDD/TTY) or headphones that can be plugged into a television, computer, or CD player.

5. Educating the family. Since the caregiver typically spends several hours a week with your loved one, he or she may pick up on some communication tips and techniques that you haven't discovered yet. The caregiver can share this advice with you, making it easier for you and your loved one to understand each other.

VISION

CHAPTER 2.1: HOW OUR EYES WORK

Much like sound, light comes to us in waves of energy. Whether or not we are able to see and make sense of these waves depends on the wavelength or the distance between the light waves. Humans can only see wavelengths that measure between 400 and 700 nanometers. This explains why we are unable to see x-rays, which average between 0.10 and 10 nanometers and radiation, which averages well over 1000 nanometers. The colors that we see also depend on wavelengths and on structures in the eye called cones, named for their cone-like shape.

The Normal Eye

The human eye is a complex structure built to capture waves of light, convert them to nerve signals, and send them to the brain for further processing and action. Each part of the eye has its own role to play in making sure that all information is transmitted properly. The following paragraphs look at specific parts of the eye and what they do.

The sclera, constructed of tough, protective tissue, covers the white part of the eye and hosts blood vessels that help nourish the eye.

The cornea rests just outside the colored part of the eye. It gathers and focuses light that will eventually be used by the brain to develop images.

The iris is the colored part of the eye, the part people refer to when they say something like, and "Your mother has the bluest eyes..." The iris, however, doesn't solely serve an aesthetic purpose. It is the home for muscles that control the way the pupil responds to light. The pupil is the dark center of the iris. It is actually an opening that allows the light gathered by the cornea to reach the lens. The pupil is very sensitive to light, contracting when there is too much light available and expanding when dark conditions make it hard to see.

The lens is a clear disc located directly behind the pupil and the iris. Its job is to focus the light rays it receives onto the retina. The lens is suspended in the eye by tough fibers attached to muscle, which subtly alter the shape of the lens to compensate for distance.

The vitreous body makes up what many people think of as the "ick" part of the eye. It is a sac filled with a clear, jelly-like substance that gives the eye its shape and provides the lubrication the eye needs to keep healthy. It is also what provides that uneasy squishy feeling when you push in on your eye. (Note: Don't push on your eye.) Light can easily penetrate the vitreous body and strike the retina.

The retina is located at the very back of the eyeball. It contains two significant building blocks called rods and cones that are sensitive to light. The rods do not detect color, but give us an object's shape and form. The cones detect and combine red, yellow and blue. They mix and match these primary colors to create every color the eye is capable of seeing.

Once these light waves have been processed, the retina transforms them to nerve signals and passes them along to the optic nerve, which then carries this information to the visual cortex in the occipital lobe of the brain.

The visual cortex is the part of the brain that actually transforms light patterns into the images that constitute what we think of as sight. It also helps us categorize and make judgments about the things we see. For instance, most of us can immediately recognize the difference between a beach ball and a cat. We also immediately know the difference between a purring kitten and a snarling mountain lion. Depending on what we see, the brain teaches us to react accordingly.

The eye, like the ear, is an extremely complex structure. In order for it to function as it should, all parts must be in working order.

As we get older, though, certain parts of our eyes—and at times parts of our brains—may stop working as reliably. The next chapter examines some of these problems with the eyes that we may experience as we age.

CHAPTER 2.2: COMMON VISION PROBLEMS

As we reach our 40s and 50s, our eyes undergo changes that affect our vision. Although many of these potential changes are easy to compensate for and have little impact on our lives, other more serious conditions can lead to permanent vision loss or blindness.

This chapter looks at eye problems that occur as we age and discusses the causes and effective treatments.

Presbyopia

Presbyopia usually begins around the age of 40. It involves a slow thickening and loss of flexibility of the lens of the eye. The result is a decreased ability to see small print or objects that you are holding close to your eyes such as needlework or crafts.

Most people with presbyopia cope by wearing bifocals—also known as progressive additional lenses or PALs—if they already have corrective lenses for another condition. If they do not require any other eyesight correction, they can use inexpensive reading glasses to magnify small or close objects and bring them into better focus.

Cataracts

According to AllAboutVision.com, more than 2.2 million Americans over the age of 40 suffer from cataracts. The National Coalition for Vision Health in Canada estimates that about 2.5 Canadians currently have cataracts, and that number continues to grow each year as the population ages. Cataracts are a cloudy buildup of protein clusters that partially cover the lens of the eye. This prevents light from shining through the lens to the retina and results in impaired vision.

Most types of cataracts form so slowly that you may not even be aware that your vision is declining. Over-exposure to ultraviolet light and diabetes appear to be two significant risk factors for cataracts. Once an eye doctor has diagnosed cataracts, they can usually be surgically removed, although they may grow back and require further surgery.

Because corrective cataract surgery is not available in many developing countries, cataracts are the most common cause of blindness worldwide.

Glaucoma

Glaucoma occurs when there is a buildup of fluid pressure inside the eye. This increased pressure blocks the flow of fluids and nutrients between the cornea and the lens and between the lens and the retina. Glaucoma has no outward symptoms and therefore may not be discovered until it has caused permanent damage to the eye.

Most eye doctors recommend a thorough eye exam including tests to measure the pressure inside the eye (intraocular pressure or IOP) at least once every two years. People in higher risk categories for glaucoma, such as older African-Americans, are encouraged to undergo testing at least once every 12 months.

Eye drops to lower fluid pressure are the most commonly prescribed treatment for glaucoma. Other types of treatment include oral medication and surgery.

Glaucoma is a leading cause of blindness for seniors in North America.

Age-Related Macular Degeneration
Age-related macular degeneration (AMD) is the most common cause of blindness for Americans over the age of 65. AMD affects the macula, or the part of the retina that is required for central vision. The most common symptom of AMD is blurring or cloudiness at the center of one's visual field. Peripheral vision usually remains clear.

There are two types of AMD: dry and wet macular degeneration. Dry macular degeneration is the most common type. Doctors don't know what causes it, but it is the result of the slow breakdown of retinal tissue. There are no treatments approved by the Food and Drug Administration for dry macular degeneration, although some research suggests that vitamins A, C, and E may slow the progression.

Wet macular degeneration occurs when new blood vessels that don't belong on the retina form. These new vessels are usually paper-thin and leak blood and fluids onto the surrounding tissue, resulting in permanent loss of vision. The FDA has approved a few medications aimed at stopping the abnormal growth of blood vessels for the treatment of wet macular degeneration.

Diabetic Retinopathy

Diabetic retinopathy occurs when the cells in the retina are damaged. Typically, it begins when blood vessels swell and deprive the retina of oxygen and blood. In an attempt to survive, new and abnormal blood vessels grow on the retina, a condition called proliferative retinopathy. These blood vessels are usually very weak and often break or develop tears that leak blood and fluids onto the retina, creating permanent damage and vision loss.

Diabetic retinopathy may occur in Type 1 or Type 2 diabetics. It has no warning symptoms and the only way to test for it is through a dilated eye exam. Most doctors recommend that diabetic patients undergo this exam at least once per year.

Although the exact cause of diabetic retinopathy is not known, some studies suggest that diabetics who are able to control their blood pressure, cholesterol levels, and blood glucose levels are at a lower risk for developing diabetic retinopathy than those who are not.

Once proliferative retinopathy is detected, doctors can use laser surgery to shrink abnormal blood vessels. Another treatment is a vitrectomy, a surgical procedure to remove a small amount of blood and fluid from the eye, thereby relieving pressure on the retina.

Retinal Detachment

A retinal detachment occurs when the retina is torn or pulled away from the blood vessels that nurture it. A retinal detachment can be repaired, but it must be attended to as soon as possible, because without the nourishment provided by the blood vessels, the cells in the retina will start to die.

Symptoms of retinal detachment include the following: small amounts of debris or "floaters" in the line of vision, a sudden flash of light in one eye, or shadows that obscure part of the visual field. Doctors can diagnose retinal detachment with painless tests that allow them to look deep inside the eye.

Retinal detachment has several causes including injury to or severe inflammation of the eye. Detachment in older adults, however, usually occurs because the vitreous body has collapsed or has begun leaking fluids so that it no longer holds the retina in place. Regardless of cause, detachments are usually treated through various surgical procedures.

Temporal Arteritis

Temporal arteritis is a relatively unusual condition that causes damage to the blood vessels that supply blood and oxygen to the head and neck. It is treatable and most people will eventually make a full recovery, but a rare side effect of the condition is sudden and irreversible loss of vision.

As we age, there are many conditions that may affect our eyes and make it difficult for us to see. The next chapter discusses how caregivers can help loved ones who suffer from vision loss, while allowing them to maintain as much independence as possible.

CHAPTER 2.3: COMPENSATING FOR VISION PROBLEMS

Not being able to see well is a problem that, if not dealt with proactively, can take away some or all of your loved one's independence. If the person you care for has vision problems, there are many ways you can help.

An Ounce of Prevention

Make sure your loved one receives a full eye exam at least once every 12 months. The exam should include dilation and a test for intraocular pressure. If your loved one had eye problems in the past or has a condition that is correlated with a higher risk for eye problems (diabetes, for instance), the doctor may recommend more frequent exams. Of course, if your loved one complains of sudden vision changes, he or she needs to be seen by a doctor as soon as possible.

Assistive Devices

There are several products on the market to help people who have trouble with vision. The most common are eyeglasses, either bifocals or simple reading glasses.

Because glasses are small and often have frame colors that blend in with neutral-colored furnishings, they can be easily misplaced. Getting a new pair made can be expensive, especially if your loved one loses his or her glasses several times a year.

Luckily, there are steps you can take to reduce the risk of glasses being lost. One option is to select bright-colored frames that are easy to spot. Another idea is to establish a place where your loved one always puts his glasses after removing them for bed, such as a colorful eyeglass case or a specific drawer in his bedside table. You can also purchase inexpensive, necklace-type jewelry so your loved one can wear the glasses around her neck when not in use.

No matter how diligently you try to prevent loss, it's always a good idea to keep an extra pair of glasses on hand, just in case.

Finally, make sure your loved one keeps the lenses of his or her eyeglasses clean. Spotted or stained lenses may actually hinder sight more than they help it.

Another handy, inexpensive assistive device is a simple magnifying glass, which can help your loved one see well enough to read, pay bills, and do other tasks that involve small print.

It's also a good idea to ensure that your loved one has at least one working flashlight or penlight that can help illuminate dark corners or hard-to-see-into drawers and cabinets.

Some older people with vision problems derive benefit from audio devices such as clocks that announce the date and time at the push of a button and voice activated health tools, such as blood-glucose meters that speak the test results. Other seniors, however, may have trouble getting used to this new technology and find it more annoying than helpful. Talk to your loved one about his or her preferences.

Super-sized devices, such as a television remote control that can be two or three times the normal size, or phones with a large base and keypad, can be handy for a person who has trouble reading small numbers.

If the person for whom you are providing care loves books but is losing his or her ability to read, check with your local library about signing up for books on tape/CD or books for the blind. Most states have programs that allow you to borrow the audio device and the books at no charge.

Adequate Lighting

Next to getting assistive devices, the best thing you can do for your loved one is to ensure adequate lighting in his or her home. You may need to add extra overhead lights to dark areas where falls commonly occur such as stairwells or walk-in closets.

It's also a good idea to go to a discount store and stock up on longneck (aka goose neck) lamps. Place one lamp on each of your loved one's desks and tables to make it easier for your loved one to read, write, pay bills and eat.

Use Color Contrast

Use sharp color contrasts to make dangerous locations such as a stairwell more obvious and to draw attention to objects that your loved one loses frequently. A black handrail against a white wall, for instance, is much easier to see than a white or silver-colored handrail against that same wall.

Of course, you don't have to restrict yourself to using just black and white. Try using colored duct tape to highlight light switches or electrical outlets, or serve your loved one's favorite meal on bright blue plates that are in sharp contrast to the brown wood of your table, for example.

Organize

The less your loved one is able to see, the more important it is for him to know exactly where every item in his home is stored.

For instance, the clean underwear should always be in the top bureau drawer, the cereal should always be in the right-hand cabinet, and so forth. As much as possible, try to adapt to the methods of organizing your loved one already uses instead of trying to make him or her learn a new method for your convenience.

To make taking medication easier and to reduce the likelihood of mistakes, purchase a large, color-coded tray, available at any pharmacy. The trays will allow you to help your loved one set up his or her medications for a week at a time. They will also make it easier for you to tell at a glance whether or not your loved one is taking medication as prescribed.

Warning! Always keep cleaning supplies, poisonous products to repel pests, and other harsh chemicals away from where food is stored. Label all such chemicals clearly with a black marker and place them in their own cupboard or drawer, away from anything that resembles food.

Driving

If your loved one's vision has declined to the point where glasses cannot provide adequate correction, he or she should not drive. Ideally, this directive will come from the eye doctor or from your state's department of motor vehicles, but sometimes you may have to be the one to actually confiscate the car keys.

It's normal for your loved one to feel hurt and angry, perhaps even a little afraid. Listen to those feelings, and then help him or her focus on other options for getting around such as friends and family members, taxis and senior transportation programs.

Money

If your loved one's declining vision makes it hard for him or her to tell one paper bill from another, help him organize his wallet so he can keep track of how much money he has on hand. You might, for instance, store each denomination in a separate compartment of the wallet, fold each type of bill a little differently, or use colored paper clips to keep the denominations together.

Outdoor Walks

For outdoor walking, or walking in unfamiliar places, the Family Caregiver Alliance recommends using the "sighted guide technique". This means that your loved one holds onto your arm just above the elbow and walks about half a pace behind you. That way, if there is an obstacle ahead, you can provide both physical support and a verbal warning ("Watch out for the step down from the curb, Mom.")

Extra Help

When you learn that your loved one's vision is poor or declining, ask the eye doctor if he or she is eligible for vision-related rehabilitation services.

Visual rehabilitation is a service for people who are blind or have limited vision. It is an intensive therapy program that teaches older adults to use assistive devices, helps them find ways to function more effectively in their homes, teaches them techniques to orient themselves in both familiar and unfamiliar surroundings, and offers support so that they can remain as independent as possible.

The first step in any visual rehabilitation program is a thorough evaluation. Your loved one will receive a detailed eye exam to see if the vision loss can be stopped or reversed.

Different specialists from the rehabilitation team will then meet with you and your loved one, usually in the home, to find out what coping mechanisms your loved one is currently using, assess safety issues, and learn how poor vision is impacting the ability to function in everyday life. For instance, one person may have no problems preparing frozen meals in the microwave, but may be unable to handle bills or correspondence. Another may suffer frequent falls as a result of tripping over clutter. A third may be afraid to move around as his or her vision deteriorates.

Once the team has identified problem areas and helped your loved one select treatment goals, they will come to his or her home on a regular basis to work on a variety of interventions including:

- Use of visual aids such as glasses
- Use of optical devices that take advantage of any vision remaining (e.g., a magnifying glass)
- Use of exercises and repetitive practice to help your loved one perform routine tasks

The visual rehabilitation team may also offer referrals to other services such as home health agencies to provide assistance around the house, mental health centers if your loved one is experiencing depression or anxiety, a representative from your loved one's bank to help determine a paperless way to handle routine bills, and a transportation service so that your loved one can get out on a regular basis.

Most visual rehabilitation teams focus on four main areas of interest:
1. Enhancing communication with friends, family and the community
2. Providing emotional support

3. Encouraging skills necessary for independent living
4. Training in the use of certain technologies and device designed to improve functioning

What about a Guide Dog?

Guide dogs, sometimes known as seeing-eye dogs, are animals trained to improve mobility for people who are blind or for those who have severe visual impairments. Seniors may be eligible for a guide dog if they meet the following criteria:

- An eye doctor documents the need for a guide dog
- The senior is independently mobile
- The senior is mentally alert enough to learn certain gestures and commands to communicate with the dog
- The senior must be able to provide routine care for the dog

Most charities that provide guide dogs have similar processes. First, the client, usually with the help of family and friends, completes a written application. If the application seems to be a match for the program, the agency sends out an expert to conduct a home interview. If the interview confirms that client would benefit from having a guide dog and is able to provide care for one, the client attends a two to four week training process. The training will teach your loved one how to communicate with the guide dog, how to provide daily routine care to keep the dog in excellent shape, and how to walk with the dog on various types of surfaces such as sidewalks, stairs, or lawns.

Family members are usually invited and often encouraged to attend training, but it will be your loved one's responsibility to independently meet each skill requirement.

To find a charity near you that provides trained guide dogs, simply go to your favorite search engine and type in "guide dogs [your location]."

It is important to be aware that because guide dogs are in high demand, agencies often have a lengthy waiting list. If you notice your loved one's eyesight declining rapidly, you may want to reach out in advance to secure a place on the waiting list.

HOW HOME CARE CAN HELP

1. Assisting with chores like filing important papers and paying bills. It may take some time to develop trust before your loved one is willing to allow someone else to help him or her with these personal tasks.

2. Encouraging regular communication with family and friends. A caregiver can help your loved one write and mail letters, make telephone calls and even send emails.

3. Reading aloud. Your loved one may enjoy having the caregiver read aloud from a favorite book.

4. Assisting with vision aids. If your loved one is constantly misplacing eyeglasses or if he or she can't figure out how to use equipment like a super-sized remote control or a talking book system, your loved one's caregiver can make sure they benefit from all the technology at their fingertips.

5. Helping with transportation and outings. Since vision-impaired adults usually can't drive, they may have a hard time getting to the store to buy food or go on a pleasant outing. A caregiver can run errands with your loved one to allow him or her chance to get out of the house.

TOUCH

CHAPTER 3.1: HOW WE PERCEIVE TOUCH

What is the largest organ of the body? If you guessed the skin, you are absolutely right! Our skin makes up about 15% of our total body weight and is in a constant state of flux, shredding and replacing more than 50 million cells each day.

The skin actually plays two roles. First it is a strong, waterproof barrier that protects the blood vessels, muscles, joints and internal organs from damage.

Second, the skin contains millions of sensors that alert us to what is happening to our bodies. Without our skin and its nerve and touch receptors, we could not tell heat from cold or a hard slap from a gentle caress. Believe it or not, we would not even be aware of our feet touching the floor as we walked.

Layers of Skin

Skin has several different layers. The three most important layers for the purposes of this book are the epidermis, the dermis and the subcutaneous tissues. The epidermis is the top layer of skin. When we look at someone's hands or face, we are actually looking at their epidermis. The epidermis consists of skin cells that have died, but have not yet flaked off the body. It also contains the substance melanin, which shields us against the ultraviolet rays of the sun by making our skin color darker, also referred to as a suntan.

The dermis lies directly below the epidermis. It is constantly generating new cells and pushing dead cells up to the epidermis.

The dermis contains several valuable structures like sweat glands and hair follicles. Most central to our discussion, the dermis is rich with nerve endings and touch receptors.

Finally, the subcutaneous tissue is the bottom level of our skin. Composed mostly of fat and connective tissue, it cushions our internal organs and protects them from harm. This tissue is also attached to our muscles and tendons. Besides basic protection, one of the most important jobs of the subcutaneous tissue is regulating body temperature.

The Somatosensory System

The somatosensory system is the vast network of nerve endings and touch receptors that are in constant communication with the brain about which action the body should take next. The human body is capable of feeling many different sensations at one time.

Take a few moments to think of all the things you can sense.

Of all the receptors the body contains, there are four that are essential to our continued survival: mechaconreceptors, thermoreceptors, proprioreceptors, and pain receptors. The mechaconreceptors sense subtle signals such as pressure, texture, vibration, and whether the body is rotating or stretching in any way. Mechaconreceptors are in action when we are in a moving car, when someone squeezes our fingers for support, or when we are petting a purring cat.

The thermoreceptors register temperature. There are both hot and cold receptors, but they can only sense temperatures in certain ranges. The cold sensors, for instance, stop registering feelings once the temperature drops below 41 degrees Fahrenheit. If you've ever felt your fingers or toes grow numb with cold, it is because their temperature has dropped to a point that can no longer be detected by the body's cold receptors. Heat receptors, on the other hand, stop sending messages to the body when the temperature rises above 113 degrees Fahrenheit, but instead of going numb, they allow pain signals to take over, urging the body to move away from the source of heat before it is damaged.

Proprioreceptors sense the position of the body in relation to yourself and your environment. They are in close touch with the tendons, muscles, and joints so we can adjust our positions as necessary. If you've ever been on a wild carnival ride and staggered out the exit door feeling disoriented and dizzy, it is because the proprioreceptors need a few seconds to register that the unexpected movement has stopped and the body is standing or sitting normally.

The most important receptors throughout the body are the pain receptors. There are three million pain receptors throughout the body. At first, this doesn't sound like a good thing. After all, who wants to feel pain? But the pain receptors are responsible for letting the brain know when your body is hurting and potentially in danger. If the pain is sharp, the brain commands us to move away from the stimulus causing the sensation. Dull pain is read as an old injury and the body sends its warning signal to keep us from causing further harm to the damaged place.

The Nervous System

The receptors in the skin communicate with the body through neurons or nerve cells. The neurons constantly receive and transmit messages from other neurons to carry important information to the brain, usually through the spinal cord. The brain analyzes the information and sends back an appropriate command such as "Take your hand away from the stove!" or "Put on gloves because it's getting cold."

The next chapter will look at age and injury-related problems that occur in the nervous system that may alter our sense of touch.

CHAPTER 3.2: COMMON PROBLEMS WITH TOUCH/FEELING

Loss of sensation is almost always the result of nerve damage that disrupts the messaging between the receptor and the brain. Damage can occur to the neurons throughout the body, the spinal cord, or the brain itself.

Peripheral Neuropathy

Damage to the nerves of the hands and feet is called peripheral neuropathy. It may be caused by problems with the circulation, vitamin deficiencies, or illnesses such as diabetes that destroy nerve endings and receptors in the dermis.

People with neuropathy usually experience tingling, pain, or numbness in the afflicted limb. Some people with neuropathy complain that their symptoms come and go quickly. A diabetic patient we worked with, for instance, said she could be walking along normally and all of the sudden not be able to feel her feet beneath her. These episodes frequently led to falls, a common problem for people with neuropathy. Another complication of peripheral neuropathy is undetected wounds to the feet. These wounds may not heal well due to decreased circulation. Infection and gangrene can then set in, sometimes making it necessary to amputate a part of the foot or the leg.

Acute Sensory Loss

Acute sensory loss involves numbness, tingling, or a complete lack of sensation in any given part of the body. It is usually the result of a stroke, a serious brain injury, a spinal cord injury, or a condition called compartment syndrome.

Compartment syndrome occurs when one part of the body's muscles or nerves are compressed so that no blood or oxygen can get through to the injured "compartment." The most common causes of compartment syndrome is a complex fracture or a crushing injury. The syndrome can be treated surgically, but the surgery must be performed quickly before the muscle tissue starts to die and become useless.

People who have had a stroke may lose all ability to feel touch, pain, temperature, or position on one or both sides of their bodies. Loss of bladder sensation and control over bladder muscles is also not uncommon. Some people who have had a stroke experience an unpleasant sensation called paresthesia, a numbness, tingling, or pain in affected body parts.

Heat and Cold

According to the Centers for Disease Control and Prevention (CDC), seniors tend to adjust poorly to sudden temperature changes. This means that your loved one can be at risk during both the hot and cold months.

Cold. Seniors tend to produce less body heat, especially those who are already sick and frail. As the temperature plummets, two things can happen to the body. The first is an abrupt increase in blood pressure which can lead to an increased risk for heart attacks, strokes, or burst aneurysms. Second, the person may develop a condition called hypothermia that causes the body temperature to drop very rapidly and places strain on the heart and lungs.

Most seniors are aware of being cold, but they worry about the expense of running the furnace. Some prefer devices like space heaters which can pose a fire hazard. If your loved one is cognitively impaired with Alzheimer's or another form of dementia, he or she may be aware of feeling cold, but not know what to do about it.

Heat. Seniors are especially vulnerable to heat for three reasons. First, as mentioned above, their bodies simply don't adjust well to extreme temperatures. Second, many seniors have chronic medical conditions that keep them from noticing extreme heat or extreme cold. Finally, some seniors are on medications that affect the way the body responds to heat.

Some seniors live in homes that are not air conditioned. Even those who do have an air conditioner may be reluctant to run it because of the cost. Your loved one may also refuse to alter his or her daily routine in response to weather conditions. Heat and exertion is an especially bad combination for aging adults. It may lead to heat cramps or muscle spasms that occur due to dehydration.

If the person does not allow him or herself to cool down, he or she may experience heat exhaustion. This occurs when the body has lost too many fluids due to perspiration. Blood flow to the skin increases, in order to regulate one's body temperature to keep it cool, which means that vital organs receive less blood. At this point, the body temperature starts to rise. The person may go into a mild state of shock and appear disinterested in what is going on around him or her. Confusion is another sign of heat exhaustion.

Untreated heat exhaustion may lead to a far more serious condition known as heat or sun stroke. At this point, the body's temperature control system has been completely overwhelmed. Sweating stops, leaving the body with no way to cool itself and the body's internal temperature can rise to 106 degrees Fahrenheit or more in a matter of minutes. A heat stroke that is not treated promptly can result in permanent brain damage or even death.

Pain

At least 20% of Americans over the age of 65 complain of chronic pain. In Canada, the percentage of seniors with complaints of chronic pain are slightly higher—25%. Among people in nursing facilities, this number climbs to 40%. This pain can have several causes. Arthritis, which occurs when one or more of the joints in the body becomes inflamed, is a common cause. Another culprit is shingles, a viral infection resulting in a tingling, stinging rash. Old injuries such as broken bones that didn't heal correctly can also cause discomfort.

Sometimes, a person who has had to have a limb amputated may experience phantom pain, or the sensation that the limb is still attached to the body and that it still hurts. Doctors are not sure why this type of pain occurs, but it seems to originate in the sensory cortex of the brain.

Another cause of pain is leftover from a life-threatening or life-limiting illness such as cancer. There are narcotic medications that help ease this kind of suffering. Doctors used to be reluctant to use them, but medical schools are now teaching graduates to treat pain more aggressively. If your loved one has a terminal illness and you are not satisfied with the level of pain control, get a second opinion or ask for a local hospice to evaluate your loved one and make comfort recommendations.

Skin Hunger

Years ago, researchers did an experiment with two groups of baby monkeys. They left the first group alone to be raised naturally by their mothers. The monkeys in the second group were removed from their mothers and placed in cages with a cloth-covered metal contraption. The contraption was wired to provide plenty of milk and the cloth was thick enough to keep the babies warm, but they were never allowed to experience a caring touch.

The monkeys in the first group thrived while those in the second group appeared under-developed, anxious and unhappy. A few even died.

Since then, further research has shown that most, if not all, humans require a certain amount of a caring touch for optimal health. Those who do not receive this touch may experience "skin hunger," a condition every bit as distressing as the longing for food and water. Or, as Dr. Bruce Rumbold, the head of the palliative care center at La Trobe University in Australia, put it, "Touch is a fundamental form of communication."

The next chapter reviews the different problems that may occur with sensation and makes suggestions about how caregivers can compensate for these issues.

CHAPTER 3.3: COMPENSATING FOR PROBLEMS WITH TOUCH/FEELING

As a caregiver, you may notice that your loved one has several issues that involve the body's abilities to feel touch and pain. There are some specific strategies you can try to help your loved one deal with these conditions.

Peripheral Neuropathy

Since the person with peripheral neuropathy is often unable to feel her feet, you need to be sure that any area where she routinely walks is clear of clutter, such as children's toys, electric cords stretched across the floor, throw rugs, or anything else that might catch under her feet and trip her.

It is also a good idea to ask your loved one's doctor if a cane or a walker might help increase their stability. If your loved one uses a walker, for instance, she might be able to grab it for support when she loses her balance and prevent a fall.

Neuropathy makes it difficult to feel your feet. A loved one who goes barefoot might easily step on a tack or a piece of broken glass without even being aware that the injury had occurred. Therefore, it is important to encourage your loved one to wear something on his feet at all times. Good choices include thick stockings with non-skid pads on the bottom, slippers (also with non-skid pads) or a pair of comfortable shoes. When your loved one gets a new pair of shoes, check his feet carefully every day to make sure that the shoes fit correctly and are not rubbing against the skin of the feet.

For that matter, if your loved one will allow it, it is a good idea to check his or her feet daily for any cuts or open sores, red spots or bruises. If your loved one has a history of peripheral neuropathy, and you find a wound on his or her foot, call the doctor promptly so that the injury can be treated before infection sets in.

Finally, make regular appointments for your loved one to see a podiatrist for a thorough foot examination and routine nail care. If your loved one has nerve damage in his feet, do not attempt to clip his nails yourself. It's easy to accidentally clip a little bit of skin and open a wound that can cause problems later.

Acute Sensory Loss

There are two types of people, who experience acute sensory loss. The first are those who experienced the loss in their younger years and are now growing older. The second are people who, as seniors, experience a catastrophic illness or injury that robs them of sensation in all or in part of their bodies.

If your loved one has a rapid onset of sensory loss, get him or her to an emergency room right away. Doctors can treat circulation problems and many types of injuries, but they must begin caring for your loved one as soon as possible for the treatments to be most effective.

If your loved one still has acute sensory loss, even after going through treatment and rehabilitation, there are some things you might want to consider about her care. First of all, more than half of people with acute sensory loss require help caring for their basic needs—eating, bathing, getting dressed, going to the restroom, etc. This level of care can be a real burden on a single caregiver, so if you don't have friends and family to help you with your loved one's needs, you might want to consider hiring a paid caregiver. This will not only give you a chance to get out and relieve your own stress, it will give your loved one a chance to socialize and engage with someone new.

Someone who is bedbound may develop bedsores no matter how carefully you treat their skin. Being immobile for long periods of time, along with the lack of good nutrition that often follows an accident or illness, makes the skin very vulnerable to breakdown. You can help minimize this problem by gently wiping your loved one's skin clean after he or she urinates or defecates. Your doctor might also suggest that you use a powder or a special kind of lotion as a moisture barrier to keep the skin as dry as possible.

As you help your loved one take care of his or her activities of daily living, look carefully at his or her skin and report any red spots or open areas to your healthcare team immediately.

Stroke Rehabilitation

According to the National Institute of Neurological Disorders and Stroke, 70,000 people in the United States and 50,000 people in Canada suffer strokes each year. Of those people, an average of 67% to 75% survive and require some type of rehabilitation.

Stroke rehabilitation should not be considered a cure. It cannot undo any brain damage the stroke has caused. What it can do is help survivors relearn some or all of their lost abilities by forging new neurological pathways in the brain—in other words, helping the healthy parts of the brain to compensate for the parts that no longer function properly.

To be the most effective, stroke rehabilitation must begin as soon as the patient has been medically stabilized from the stroke, usually within 24 to 48 hours. The first thing rehabilitation specialists want people to work on is regaining as much independent movement as possible. This involves getting the patient out of bed and into a chair as soon as it is medically safe to do so. Furthermore, people are encouraged to change position frequently, perhaps by shifting from one side to another, during the time that they are in bed. If the person is no longer able to manage any independent movement, he or she will receive a type of therapy known as passive range of motion (ROM).

Passive range of motion can be done by a physical therapist, a nurse, a nurse's aide, or even a trained family member. It involves gently contracting and stretching the muscles in the arms, legs, hands and feet.

Most people who have suffered a stroke receive their initial treatment at an inpatient rehabilitation facility. This lasts a few days to a few weeks, after which people generally continue to receive therapy at an outpatient clinic or in their own homes. You may be able to help by learning to physically assist your loved one with his or her prescribed exercise routine. You can also be a tremendous source of emotional support during what is usually a very trying time.

Rehabilitation services offer many different types of therapy to help people who have suffered sensory loss on one or both sides of their bodies. Some therapies your loved one may be exposed to include:

- Exercises to build muscle coordination and strength
- Mobility training to relearn the skill of walking

- "Constraint induced" therapy, which involves immobilizing the stronger side so that the patient is forced to use his or her weaker side
- Electrical stimulation to help weakened muscles relearn how to contract
- Robotic technology to practice and relearn repetitive motions

Rehabilitation services are also available to help with problems like receptive aphasia, or the inability to understand speech and expressive aphasia, or the inability to speak, and problems with swallowing food and liquids.

It is also standard for stroke rehabilitation patients to receive a psychological evaluation to assess their most helpful coping mechanisms and screen for problems like depression and anxiety which typically respond well to counseling and medication.

Assistive Devices for Stroke Patients

Intensive rehabilitation can be very helpful for some stroke patients, but it doesn't work for everybody. Even those who do benefit from it greatly may have a few residual deficits in their ability to feel and move. Talk with your loved one's rehabilitation team about any assistive devices that might give your loved one back some of his or her independence.

Hospital Beds. If your loved one has to spend most of his or her time in bed, ask the doctor to arrange to have a hospital bed delivered to the home. The doctor may also want to order a special kind of mattress like an air or ripple mattress, which can stimulate the skin or a rotational mattress, which turns your loved one in bed on a regular basis. All of these special mattresses can help reduce the risk of bedsores. Insurance will cover most types of hospital beds.

Wheelchairs and scooters. There are many types of wheelchairs and scooters. Some have straight backs. Some have reclining capability. Some require the patient to use his or her own strength to propel the device and others are battery operated. Your loved one's rehabilitation team can advise you about the equipment that will best help your loved one maintain the most mobility. If your loved one will be spending a large part of his or her day in the chair, ask about a gel cushion or a positioning pillow to take the pressure off the coccyx (tailbone). Again, insurance usually covers the cost of a wheelchair and, in some cases, the cost of a scooter.

Lifts. Many people who have had a stroke, even those who have not regained full mobility, are able to sit up on the bed, stand and pivot with assistance, and sit down in a wheelchair or easy chair. Some stroke sufferers, however, are never able to regain enough strength in their legs to transfer from one surface to another, even with assistance. These people may benefit from having a device like a sit-to-stand lift or a Hoyer lift in the home. Both of these lifts involve using slings to mechanically transfer your loved one between surfaces or to help support them while you cleanse the skin after incontinence. Although advertisements for some lifts suggest that the lift can be operated by only one caregiver, most hospitals and nursing homes recommend a minimum of two caregivers for a lift transfer. Talk to your loved one's rehabilitation team and see what they suggest.

If your loved one needs just a little help to get out of a seat, consider buying him or her a reclining chair with a "lift" feature. These chairs can be expensive and they are generally not covered by insurance, but they can help your loved one maintain his or her independence when it comes to standing and walking.

Other mobility aids for those less impaired include various types of canes and walkers.

Toileting Assistance. If your loved one has trouble getting to the bathroom in time, you may need to ask your rehabilitation team to order a commode for you. A commode is placed by the patient's bed so that they can transfer directly from the bed to the commode. This ease of getting to the toilet can resolve many incontinence problems. If your loved one is still able to make it to the bathroom, be sure to install grab bars that he or she can use to break a fall. Do not depend on the towel rack for this—the towel rack was not created for that purpose and will pull away from the wall if too much weight is applied to it. Many people who have strokes have trouble getting up from a sitting position, especially if the seat is very low, like most toilet seats. You can resolve this problem by buying a toilet seat riser. Most risers are about four inches tall and fit over the regular toilet seat. With the help of the grab bars mentioned earlier, your loved one may be able to toilet him or herself without assistance.

It's also a good idea to talk with your loved one's rehabilitation team about toilet wiping aids. People who have had a stroke and/or people who are significantly overweight may not be able to reach the perianal area to wipe after urination or a bowel movement. Wiping aids give the patient extra reach. Some of them are bendable, which also helps your loved one in getting at difficult to reach places.

Hygiene. There are many products to help your loved one maintain his or her hygiene such as handheld portable showers, long-handled bathing sponges, inflatable sinks for shampooing and bathing if your loved one cannot get out of bed, and foam handles that can be used to make a toothbrush or make a razor easier to grip. (Speak with your loved one's rehabilitation team before allowing them to shave him or herself.)

Getting dressed. Tools that can help your loved one get dressed include reachers to grasp far away items, long handled shoe horns (often combined with reachers), aids for fastening buttons and zippers, and kits to help you put on either regular or compression stockings.

Eating. Large-handled silverware and weighted utensils and cups can be of great help if your loved one has trouble with fine motor movements or if he or she has tremors.

Extreme Temperatures

If your loved one lives alone, making it a point to check in, especially during the extreme hot days of summer and cold days of winter is important. During cold weather, your loved one is at risk for hypothermia. Also, depending on how your loved one keeps his or her home warm, he or she may also be at risk for fire or for the inhalation of natural gas or carbon monoxide. If you go to visit your loved one on a cold day and find him or her complaining of being cold, shivering, or appearing detached and confused, wrap him or her in warm clothing, coats and blankets. Have your loved one seen by a doctor to check for injuries like frostbite, and try to arrange for him or her to stay in a heated home until the weather becomes warmer.

One man, for instance, who found he couldn't stand the cold air of the Midwest during the winter months, made arrangements to move to an assisted living facility in Florida from November through April and to live in his own home from May through October.

Heat is also a concern when dealing with the elderly. Many seniors feel chronically chilled and may not realize that the temperature is actually dangerously high. You can help by warning your loved one about heat alerts. Encourage him or her to drink plenty of fluids (unless the doctor has placed your loved one on a fluid restriction—if this is the case talk to your loved one's doctor), stay out of the sun and in shaded areas when possible and wear lightweight clothing.

You can also encourage your loved one to avoid moving around during the heat of the day. If he or she has an air conditioner, encourage him or her to use it when temperatures start to feel unbearable. If they do not have an air conditioner, try to help him or her find alternatives such as moving in with a family member until the heat lets up or spending days in places that have air conditioning like senior centers, shopping malls, movie theaters and libraries.

Pain

It's always distressing when someone you care about is in pain, especially if the type of pain your loved one has is hard to treat, like arthritis pain. Still, it is important for you to know that your loved one is having this symptom, so make sure to ask specifically if he or she is in any pain. Sometimes, you may be able to tell that your loved one is hurting because he is in a foul mood or she won't participate in her favorite activities. You may also see signs of pain like wincing upon movement, "guarding" the painful area, walking much more slowly than usual, or flinching when a certain spot is touched.

If you have concerns about your loved one's pain control, consider having him or her evaluated at a pain center or clinic. Talk to your loved one's doctor before you start a regimen of over the counter pain medicine. Not all over the counter medications are safe for every patient, especially if that patient is taking other medications or has other medical conditions.

If your loved one suffers from arthritis, encourage him or her to engage in gentle movement as much as possible. For example, take a short walk or go to a community center for a dip in the heated pool. You may even want to check out a yoga class specifically for older adults. For instance, Silver Age Yoga, based in San Diego, CA, is based on principles of geriatric science emphasizing health enhancing benefits designed specifically for seniors so that they can safely participate in the exercises at their level of comfort. There are similar senior yoga studios and certification courses throughout North America. It may be hard to encourage your loved one with arthritis to move because in the short term movement hurts, but in the long-term, movement will ease the pain and keep the body limber as it strengthens the muscles that support the joints.

If your loved one is uncomfortable, you might also try using warm towels or a towel wrapped around a baggie of ice to help soothe the pain away. Another common tactic that helps ease the pain is gently elevating the sore limb.

Finally, try distracting your loved one by watching a favorite television program with him or playing some of his favorite music. Another method of distraction is to share favorite memories. You might even try engaging your loved one in a friendly debate—when we're busy vigorously defending our point of view, we don't have nearly as much time to notice pain.

What to Expect from a Pain Management Clinic

A pain management clinic uses a multidisciplinary team made up of doctors, psychologists, physiatrists, physical and occupational therapists, and sometimes holistic healers like acupuncturists or massage therapists to diagnose and treat chronic pain. Unlike acute pain, which is the type of pain you experience if you scrape your knee, chronic pain often has no apparent physical cause, but can be just as severe. Because it lasts for months or even years, it can destroy a person's quality of life if not addressed.

Pain management clinics typically combine several interventions to try to control the pain. Some of the treatments typically used at pain clinics include:

- Over-the-counter medications such as Tylenol or Advil
- Corticosteroids, or prescription drugs that help relieve inflammation
- Opioids, or narcotic-based pain medications—doctors typically steer clear of opioids as a long-term pain reliever because of addiction risk
- Antidepressants—some tricyclic antidepressants ease pain and help with falling asleep
- Injections—corticosteroids or local anesthesia may be injected to relieve inflammation and muscle spasms
- Nerve blocks—injections of local anesthetics block sensation from a targeted group of nerve cells
- Individual exercise programs to help maintain flexibility and build muscle strength
- Whirlpool therapy
- Deep muscle massage for relaxation and to ease muscle spasms
- TENS unit—painless electrical treatment used to stimulate certain nerves.
- Acupuncture

- Counseling and relaxation techniques
- Surgery (e.g., to relieve a spinal injury or to replace an arthritic knee)

Skin Hunger

Most people require some form of caring touch to function well physically and emotionally. If you suspect your loved one is hungry for touch, here are some ideas you can try:

- Offer hugs, kisses, and cuddles on a regular basis if your loved one is receptive to that kind of touch.
- Gently take your loved one's hand while you are talking or watching television.
- When you provide physical care to your loved one, do so gently and lovingly, making sure to respect his or her dignity.
- Offer to wash or brush your loved one's hair.
- Offer to help your loved one shave.
- Give your loved one a manicure (Do not offer a pedicure if your loved one has diabetes or a history of peripheral neuropathy).
- Sit close together to share a book, newspaper, or set of favorite pictures.
- If your loved one has acute sensory loss, make sure to touch a part of his or her body that he or she can feel.
- Massage your loved one's scalp, neck, or shoulders.
- If your loved one likes animals, consider getting a dog or a cat—not only is petting an animal soothing, pets are also a great source of unconditional love.

If you're not used to touching your loved one, some of these suggestions might sound pretty challenging. However, when you try them, you're likely to find that they bring comfort to both you and your loved one. If you are unsure whether the attention is welcomed or not, simply ask. For example, you can say: "I'd love to give you a hug before I go. Would that be all right?", "Your shoulders are so tense! Let me rub them for a few minutes and see if we can make that headache better.", or "Mom, your nail polish is a little chipped. Let me put on a new coat for you."

Our body is designed to be attuned to every touch, nuance, or change of pressure. Even if your loved one has a significant amount of sensory loss, you can still use the sensation of touch to communicate reassurance and affection.

HOW HOME CARE CAN HELP

1. Providing caring touch. A caregiver can offer hugs, hand-holding, massages and gentle personal care assistance. Assisting with mobility. Many people, who walk with the help of a cane or a walker, forget to use them. A caregiver can provide reminders and help your loved one keep track of assistive devices. He or she can also use equipment like a gait belt or a lift to help your loved one get from the bed to a chair.

2. Ensuring halls and walkways are free of clutter. The caregiver can check for things that might trip your loved one like an electric cord stretched across a highway, a grandchild's toys, or even long pieces of oxygen tubing that can get twisted around the feet.

3. Assisting with exercise and range of motion. If your loved one is awake, your home care worker can encourage him or her to go for a short walk each day or to perform gentle

exercise routines like yoga. Even if your loved one is bedbound, the worker can still gently stretch and contract the muscles to maintain flexibility.

4. Checking skin. If your caregiver helps bathe your loved one, ask him or her to keep an eye on your loved one's skin and let you know immediately if they notice any bruises, cuts, or red spots on pressure points like the heels or base of the spine.

SMELL

CHAPTER 4.1: HOW OUR NOSES WORK

Compared to the ear and they eye, the basic structure of the nose is less complex. It consists of two holes or nostrils separated by a thin wall of cartilage called the septum. Behind the nose are the nasal passages and the nasal cavity that connects the nose to the back of the throat.

The nose plays an important part in moving warm, moist, filtered air into the lungs. It is also, of course, responsible for detecting different scents or odors. At the top of the nasal passageway, behind the nose, sits a group of millions of neurons or nerve cells. Despite their vast numbers, they only take up a postage stamp sized space. These neurons are covered with fine hairs called cilia. Specific types of scent molecules bond with specific cilia, which triggers the attached neuron to fire off a message to the brain. The olfactory bulb of the brain then interprets the electrical impulse as scent. Most human beings can detect up to 10,000 different smells—and that's not even a tenth of what some animals are able to detect.

There are two different ways that scent molecules reach the neurons (sometimes referred to as scent receptors). The first is through inhalation. Scent molecules are composed of lightweight chemicals that evaporate quickly. Some objects, such as roses, give off many scent molecules. Others, such as steel, give off none at all. That is why some substances, including steel, have no distinctive smell.

Chewing food also releases aroma molecules into the nasal passageway where they can be captured by the cilia. Smell is a vital part of our sense of taste (see Section 5). Thus, problems with being able to sense smells can also lead to problems with the appetite.

Importance of Smell

Our sense of smell is important for many reasons. It is often our first warning sign that something is wrong. For example, we usually smell smoke before we see a fire or feel the heat of the flames. Also, rotten or poisonous substances usually smell so awful we aren't even tempted to put them in our mouths.

Another reason we need the sense of smell is because that it, more than any other sense, is linked to the limbic system. The limbic system sits at the base of our brains. Its sole purpose is survival. Unlike the frontal cortex, it has no sense of right or wrong, appropriate or inappropriate behavior. Some scientists call it the "animal" part of our brains. The limbic system processes strong memories and feelings and has no sense of time or place. That is why a whiff of perfume on a passerby may send you hurtling back into memories of a painful breakup and why walking into a bakery may make you feel as if you are helping your grandmother bake bread in her kitchen.

Like the other senses, the sense of smell usually becomes weak with age. The next chapter will look at common issues that affect the ability to process and recognize different scents.

CHAPTER 4.2: COMMON PROBLEMS WITH SMELL

According to the National Institute on Aging and the National Institutes of Health, nearly 25% of Americans over age 55 have presbyosmia, or age-related problems sensing smell. About 33% of people over the age of 80 suffer from this condition.

There is no specific cause known for presbyosmia, and doctors consider it irreversible. There are, however, several lifestyle factors that can reverse the loss of the sense of smell. Smoking, allergies, chronic colds, and chronic sinus infections are all common culprits. Some medications are also known to interfere with the sense of smell. In most cases, discontinuing the offending medication takes care of the problem.

Most aging adults with presbyosmia report that, although their sense of smell has become somewhat dull, they can still make out some distinctive odors.

Anosmia

Anosmia occurs when a person loses his or her sense of smell altogether. Some causes of anosmia include severe and chronic sinus disease, a blockage such as a tumor or a foreign object in the nasal passageway, viral infections, or head trauma, resulting in damage to the olfactory bulb of the brain.

Phantosmia

Another problem with smell, phantosmia, occurs when a person believes he or she smells something even if there is nothing in the environment able to cause the smell. Phantosmia often indicates a problem with the temporal lobe of the brain such as seizures, migraines, or even a tumor.

Certain respiratory infections can also lead to phantosmia.

Phantosmia is often reported by people who believe that a deceased loved one has come back to visit them. ("I smelled the lotion my mother always used on her hands" or "I smelled lilacs like my grandfather used to grow in the garden.") These episodes of phantosmia rarely come to the attention of doctors, both because they tend to be one-time events and because the person who experiences the phantom smell usually finds it comforting rather than distressing.

Although losing one's sense of smell may not seem like a big problem compared with losing one's eyesight, a diminished sense of smell can carry some real physical risks for your loved one. As a caregiver, there are some issues you need to be aware of, which we will discuss in the next chapter

CHAPTER 4.3: COMPENSATING FOR PROBLEMS WITH SMELL

Do you think losing the sense of smell is merely an irritant? Think again. A study at Rush University Medical Center in Chicago found that senior citizens who could identify at least 11 out of 12 everyday odors were likely to live several years longer than those who identified six odors or fewer. These results remained the same even when researchers factored out age, health status, and cognitive conditions like dementia.

Early Warning System Disabled
There are several reasons why a reduced sense of smell can hasten death. First, people who can't smell aren't able to detect warning signals like the odor of smoke or natural gas. Therefore, if your loved one has dulled sense of smell, make sure to install smoke detectors throughout his or her home. If money is an issue, the fire department in most communities will provide and even install free smoke detectors to anyone, who requests them.

If feasible, you may also want to consider helping your loved one switch from natural gas to electricity. This avoids the risk of inadvertently inhaling toxic fumes in the event of a gas leak.

If your loved one doesn't pick up on smells, he or she may accidentally eat food that has gone bad. Use a black marker to clearly label the food in your loved one's refrigerator with the expiration date. Dispose of that food after the expiration date passes.

Some older people, especially those who grew up during the Depression may protest at the idea of throwing away "good food." If this is an issue that upsets your loved one, try buying very small quantities of perishable food at a time so that less is wasted. It may be wise to wait until your loved one is involved in an activity in another part of the house before cleaning out the refrigerator.

Embarrassing Odors

Most of us have trouble getting an accurate idea of how our bodies smell. If your loved one's sense of odor is diminished, he or she may fail to recognize an important giveaway of poor personal hygiene, bad odor. Some people, who become incontinent, for instance, don't smell the odor of urine. They may wear soiled clothes or bathe infrequently. Some older men and women use too much cologne or perfume. Because they can't smell the overwhelming scent, they assume others can't either.

If bathing or showering is physically difficult for your loved one, consider hiring a private duty aide who can drop by a few times a week to help them freshen up.

If your loved one is capable of bathing on his or her own but simply doesn't like to do so, it may help to plan regular outings during the week. These outings can include activities like going to church, eating at a nice restaurant, volunteering at a Goodwill store, or merely taking a pleasant walk in the park. Make bathing a part of a ritual before you leave the house.

Finally, if your efforts at tact fail, you may need to have a kind, but honest, discussion with your loved one about the need for regular baths and clothing changes. Emphasize that you are not trying to insult them, but that you know he or she wouldn't want to be embarrassed in public.

HOW HOME CARE CAN HELP

1. Checking to make sure that all the food in the refrigerator is fresh. Since your loved one may not be able to smell spoiled food, it is important to dispose of anything that should no longer be eaten.

2. Check for odd smells in the house. A caregiver can detect potentially dangerous odors that your loved one cannot. Some odors to be especially aware of are the rotten-egg smell of a gas leak, the harsh smell of any chemicals that might be leaking, the smell of urine or feces that suggests your loved one may be have had an accident, and any pet-related odors.

3. Assisting with personal hygiene. A home health care worker is generally pretty adept at making their clients feel comfortable with taking showers and baths. This can spare your loved one the embarrassment of venturing out in public with an offensive body odor.

4. Experimenting with different smells to enhance the taste of food. Since a large part of taste is based on our sense of smell, difficulties with smell may cause a reduced desire for food and poor appetite. The home care worker can work with your loved one to see if there are any foods that still smell appealing.

5. Checking fire alarm batteries on a regular basis. Most people first become aware of a house fire because they smell smoke. If your loved one cannot smell smoke, it is vital to make sure that all the fire alarms in the house are in good condition. Fire departments typically suggest checking batteries whenever daylight savings time begins and ends. Your home care worker can help with this chore and let you know if something seems to be wrong with one of the alarms. The fire department in your city will usually replace broken or malfunctioning alarms at no cost to you.

TASTE

CHAPTER 5.1: HOW OUR TASTE BUDS WORK

The most important thing to remember about the sense of taste is that it is highly dependent upon the sense of smell. In fact, the human brain is only capable of identifying five specific flavors: sweet, sour, salty, bitter, and savory.

Our experience of taste starts when saliva combines with food to break it down chemically. The human mouth contains about 10,000 taste buds. Most are found in the bumps on your tongue (papillae), although there are a few taste buds located in the palate and in the throat.

Taste buds are called direct chemoreceptors because they must physically make contact with the chemicals in food to trigger a message to the brain. This contrasts with the other senses, for example, vision, that allow us to become aware of an object without physically touching it.

After the food in the mouth is broken down into chemicals by being chewed and mixed with saliva, these chemicals are captured by fine hairs called microvilli on the taste buds. At the same time, chewing also releases aroma molecules, which are processed by the neurons at the top of the nasal passageway.

Once the chemicals in the food come into contact with the microvilli, the taste buds convert the chemical signals into electrical impulses which are then transmitted to the gustatory cortex of the brain for additional processing and interpretation.

The sense of taste is pretty uncomplicated, but as with all the other senses, aging and lifestyle can take their toll. The next chapter looks at different problems that may occur with the sense of taste and examines some of the most common causes.

CHAPTER 5.2: COMMON PROBLEMS WITH TASTE

According to the National Institutes of Health, each year more than 200,000 seniors go to their doctors for problems with taste. Many of these cases end up being traced back to an issue with smell instead.

There are four basic categories of taste problems. The first, phantom taste perception, occurs when a person experiences an unpleasant taste of food even if there is currently nothing in their mouth. Some foods are known for leaving an unappealing aftertaste. Other times, the problem can be traced back to poor dental hygiene. Brushing your teeth or rinsing your mouth with a mild or diluted mouthwash usually takes care of the problem.

Hypogeusia, or a dullness of the sense of taste, is an issue that usually originates because of a problem with the sense of smell. Other causes may include a reduced number of taste buds due to the aging process, radiation therapy that targets the head, neck, or throat, coming into contact with chemicals that damage the taste buds, taking certain medications, and having a zinc deficiency.

Ageuisa refers to the inability to taste any flavors at all. This is a rare condition that is usually related to genetic problems or a severe injury to the back of the head where the gustatory cortex lies.

Finally, dysgeusia occurs when a familiar flavor is distorted into something unpleasant. A person may find, for instance, that once-favorite foods taste metallic or spoiled. This problem is often related to poor oral hygiene. Also, some medications can also make familiar food taste strange and unappetizing.

The worst thing about problems with taste is that they can lead to poor dietary habits. The next chapter offers some suggestions on resolving problems with nutrition.

CHAPTER 5.3: COMPENSATING FOR PROBLEMS WITH TASTE

Some geriatric experts believe that up to half of all older adults don't get adequate nutrition. There are many factors that play a part in this problem. For one, people on a fixed income may not be able to afford nutritious foods. Others may lack reliable transportation to get to a grocery store. But it is also an undeniable fact that people who no longer enjoy food are likely to eat less of it. They may also choose to eat only items that still taste good (e.g., sweets) in place of a balanced diet.

If your loved one complains about changes in his or her sense of taste, your first stop should be the doctor's office. A doctor can help determine whether the real issue is smell, taste, or a combination of both. A doctor can also see if any of your loved one's medications might be causing the problem and examine them for allergies or chronic upper respiratory infections that could play a role.

It is also a good idea for your loved one to have a dental checkup, since rotting teeth, gum disease, and poor oral hygiene can all play a part in making food undesirable.

If, after these treatments, your loved one's sense of taste does not improve, here are a few ideas that may help him or her get adequate nutrition:

- Encourage your loved one to try new things. If he won't eat his old favorite foods, suggest some nutritious alternatives such as fresh fruit or vegetables or a different kind of meat than they are used to eating. The new foods may be more appealing for your loved one than the old foods that suddenly don't taste the same.

- Hire a caregiver to help with meal preparation. If food no longer tastes good, your loved one may simply decide to stop cooking for herself. A caregiver can work with your loved one to find ways to enhance the flavoring of favorite foods to making eating enjoyable again.

- Enhance the flavor and scent of food by adding rich sauces and heart-healthy seasonings.

- Add some variety to your loved one's diet by providing food of different textures and temperatures. Even if he doesn't taste much, a cup of hot soup followed by a dish of frozen yogurt may look appetizing.

- Encourage healthy snacking instead of three large meals a day. Make sure your loved one always has plenty of her favorite nutritious snack foods on hand.

- Avoid "empty" calories, or foods that are high in calories while offering little in the way of nutrition.

- Avoid alcohol. Too much alcohol can affect the way things taste. Also, a person whose stomach is full of alcohol is more likely to make bad self-care decisions and skip meals.

- Talk to a doctor about supplements. Some doctors think using supplemental shakes or protein bars is a great idea to slip in some extra nutrition, while others are less enthusiastic. Find out what your doctor thinks before encouraging your loved one to take supplements.

- Make sure your loved one brushes his teeth or regularly cleans his dentures.

HOW HOME CARE CAN HELP

1. Preparing meals. People who have trouble tasting food are unlikely to cook on their own. Therefore, having a home care worker who can prepare meals can help ensure that your loved one gets adequate nutrition. The home care worker can also experiment with your loved one to find foods that still taste good.

2. Encouraging eating and socializing. Eating is a social ritual in North America. We get together not only to nourish our bodies but to connect with the people we care about. Even if your loved one isn't interested in food, he or she may take a few bites out of habit during a spirited conversation.

3. Maintaining oral hygiene. A caregiver can help your loved one clean his or her dentures and brush his or her teeth. This can help remove the unpleasant aftertastes some foods leave behind.

4. Keeping track of dentures. If your loved one suffers from vision problems or cognitive deficiencies like dementia, dentures might tend to disappear. Sometimes your loved one will take them out and forget where he or she placed them. Other times, especially if the dentures are becoming uncomfortable, your loved one will simply throw them away. And then there's the story of a nursing home resident, who proudly showed the nurse how she was soaking her dentures... in the toilet bowl. A caregiver can keep an eye on dentures and make sure they end up in the correct containers.

5. Monitoring weight. Ask your caregiver to coax your loved one onto the scales at least once a month. If the aide reports that your loved one is losing weight, it's time for a visit to the doctor to discuss options that might exist to improve his or her appetite.

CHAPTER 6: DEMENTIA AND THE FIVE SENSES

People are often confused about how Alzheimer's disease relates to dementia and why the two terms are used interchangeably.

Dementia is a cluster of symptoms that include poor judgment, memory loss, inability to complete simple tasks, and difficulty orienting yourself in your environment. (This is why so many dementia patients ask to go home even when they are at home.)

There are many causes of dementia. A few, like medication interactions, malnutrition, and depression can be reversed, so that the sufferer returns to his or her previous level of functioning. Most types of dementia, however, are caused by diseases that cannot be reversed. Alzheimer's disease is the most common cause of dementia, closely followed by vascular dementia or dementia caused by a series of strokes. Other types of dementia causes include Lewy body dementia, complications from Parkinson's, and Pick disease. Because Alzheimer's disease is the most common cause of irreversible dementia, it is often used interchangeably with the symptoms it causes.

The relationship between dementia and the five senses is quite complex. On the one hand, dementia is known to cause sensory problems, especially issues with vision and smell. On the other hand, studies show that some types of sensory loss in the elderly place senior citizens at a higher risk for developing dementia.

Hearing

Hearing loss may be mistaken for dementia because it can lead to many of the same symptoms: social withdrawal, inability to follow conversations, and answering questions inappropriately. Assistive devices like hearing aids and cochlear implants usually resolve these problems.

Within the past few years, however, researchers have noticed a disturbing trend: According to a study published in the Archives of Neurology, seniors who have mild to moderate hearing loss are nearly two times more likely to develop dementia than seniors whose hearing is normal. Seniors with severe hearing loss are five times more likely to develop Alzheimer's or a related condition.

It isn't clear from the current research whether hearing loss actually causes dementia or whether both dementia and hearing loss are caused by another, unknown factor. It is also unknown whether getting hearing loss treated can stave off the onset of dementia.

When your loved one suffers from both dementia and hearing loss, it is especially important to stand directly in front of him and make eye contact before speaking. Otherwise, your voice may seem to come out of nowhere, which can be frightening for people with dementia.

When you do speak, don't yell. Speak slowly and clearly. Use short sentences with gestures if appropriate, and give your loved one plenty of time to understand what you said so they can formulate a response. It is not at all uncommon for a full minute or more to pass between the time you ask a question or make a statement and the time your loved one responds. Be as patient as you can and try to avoid rushing to provide answers for your loved one. Remember, even though we live in a culture that dreads pauses in conversation, a few minutes of silence is not a bad thing.

Vision

As is true with hearing, a study published a few years ago by the American Journal of Epidemiology revealed that elders with untreated vision problems are more likely to develop dementia than those with normal vision. The key word in this study is untreated. Adults who received treatments for eye conditions like glaucoma and cataracts significantly reduced their risk of developing dementia.

Vision changes may cause dementia, but they are certainly also an effect. Many diseases of the brain that result in dementia can lead to "visual mistakes", such as perceiving that the people on the television screen are actually in the room, misidentifying a health care worker as a family member, or having hallucinations (seeing something that isn't there).

Lewy body dementia frequently causes vivid hallucinations that seem to center around seeing young children. Some people find these visions upsetting ("Get that kid out of here! She doesn't belong in my room!"), while others find them soothing ("I just love watching that little girl play with her dolls.")

Try not to allow yourself to get drawn into an argument about whether or not what your loved one sees is "real." An honest, respectful response is, "I don't see that, but I believe that you do." Sometimes the best way to handle visual mistakes is to try to step into your loved one's reality.

One woman, for instance, lived at home with the assistance of a 24/7 home aide. Every afternoon the woman became very upset, started crying, and begged the home care worker to "call the police to make those people stop fighting."

After thinking about it, the caregiver realized that the woman's anxiety increased whenever she watched a talk show known for its violent verbal and physical outbursts. The caregiver found that all she had to do to calm her patient was to face the television and say firmly, "There's no arguing allowed in this house. You all have to go home." Then she turned the television off and quickly involved her patient in another activity. Before long, she altered their daily schedule so that they were not at home when the upsetting program aired. The woman never said anything about calling the police again.

People with dementia, especially people with Alzheimer's disease, also suffer from a lack of perception. For example, they may have a decreased awareness of the different colors, or they may have trouble perceiving something that is set against a background of similar color (e.g., plain mashed potatoes served on a white plate). They may also have trouble perceiving motion, for instance, not being able to calculate how quickly an object is moving towards them.

Another common problem is depth perception. If your kitchen floor has a black and white pattern, for instance, your loved one may avoid walking on the dark tiles because to him or her, they look like holes in the floor. Lack of depth and spatial perception may also lead to your loved one "missing" the seat of a chair or the edge of the couch when he or she tries to sit down. This can result in embarrassing and possibly injury-causing falls.

If you see evidence that your loved one is having trouble with perception, especially motor perception, talk to their general practitioner or eye doctor. Ask him or her to instruct your loved one to stop driving. If the doctor isn't helpful, you can also call the Department of Motor Vehicles in your area and request that your loved one be required to take a driving test. If he or she fails the test, the DMV will revoke their driver's license.

Touch

The sense of touch is generally not altered by dementia as long as your loved one is not affected by another medical condition such as stroke or diabetic neuropathy.

In fact touch, or tactile stimulation as therapists call it, can be an excellent way to soothe and communicate with someone, who has dementia. If you are helping your loved one dress, for example, tactile cues can make the process much easier. Saying, "Mom, put your left arm through the sleeve", while gently placing a hand on her left arm, can help give her a much better idea of what you want.

There are other ways to use tactile stimulation. In the section about touch, we discussed the concept of skin hunger and how humans need a certain amount of physical closeness. Using passive stimulation means touching your loved one in a gentle, non-threatening way. This includes holding hands, cuddling up to watch television, gentle massaging the scalp, neck, and shoulders, or helping your loved one style her hair or paint her nails.

Active tactile stimulation encourages the person with dementia to touch and work with objects of different textures. You loved one might enjoy kneading Play-Doh or non-toxic modeling clay. You might also ask him or her to help you arrange flowers from your garden or to fold warm, soft towels. Certain children's books provide all sorts of different textures to touch and talk about, and many dementia patients love going through these books over and over.

The last issue relating to dementia and touch is pain. Until just a few years ago, most medical professionals believed, and taught, that people with dementia did not feel pain as sharply as people, without dementia. Brain scan studies, however, show that the opposite is true. People with dementia do feel pain, perhaps even more acutely than their unimpaired counterparts. The complicating factor is that people with dementia often aren't able to explain that they are hurting or describe the pain. Some people with dementia will deny pain if asked, even if they are obviously feeling discomfort.

Because you are with your loved one on a regular basis, you are in the best position to observe behavior changes that might suggest pain. You may see some of the following signs:

- Crying for no apparent reason
- Increased irritability
- Wincing or grimacing
- Calling out, moaning, or groaning with movement
- Guarding a part of the body, or trying to protect it so that it isn't touched
- Suddenly using the non-dominant hand for daily tasks
- Restlessness
- Signs of injury or compromised health such as bruises, burns, cuts, or bedsores

If you suspect your loved one is in pain, contact his or her doctor for immediate evaluation and treatment.

Smell

As with at least two other senses, losing one's sense of smell may be a predictor of cognitive decline. A study in the Archives of General Psychiatry found that a deficient sense of smell is often a precursor to mild cognitive impairment (MCI). MCI typically means that a person has some memory and thinking impairments that are not severe enough to disrupt his or her life. Over time, MCI often progresses to full-blown dementia.

The study scored people on the number of common smells they were able to recognize. Those in the lowest 25% were more than twice as likely to develop MCI as those in the top 25%.

It is important to realize that your loved one's sense of smell may be significantly impaired. However, if their condition is reversible, you may be able to use familiar aromas to bring back happy and comforting memories. Most people, for instance, respond positively to the scent of baked goods, flowers, or fresh laundry.

You may also want to see how your loved one reacts to scents used in aromatherapy. Lavender, for example, is said to induce relaxation and promote mental balance while rosemary can stimulate the mind and improve one's mood.

Taste

Because dementia is so strongly linked with a declining sense of smell, and because much of what we taste depends on our sense of smell, many people with dementia lose all or most of their sense of taste.

This can lead to apathy about food, weight loss, and malnutrition. It can also lead a dementia patient to put inappropriate items in his or her mouth, mistaking them for food. One man with dementia, for example, would finish his morning coffee each day and then eat the Styrofoam cup. His family and caregivers learned to swoop down and take the cup out of his hands the moment the coffee was gone. The man's youngest sister finally supplied the missing piece of the puzzle. Because her brother had always loved to eat soup out of bread bowls, he was probably mistaking the pliable Styrofoam for bread. The man's family brought him some unbreakable plastic cups to drink from and the problem disappeared.

Some people may try to put pretty items in their mouth like a flower, greeting card, or stuffed animal. Others attempt to eat non-edible food items that tend to have a strong, pleasant smell like perfume, shampoo, or hand lotion. It is important to be aware of these tendencies and to keep non-food items that seem to tempt your loved one out of his or her reach.

You may also notice that your loved one uses excessive condiments on foods to try to strengthen the taste. Although it is not the healthiest behavior, it may not be worth the effort required to prevent. Obviously, if your loved one has a heart condition, you don't want him or her covering food in salt; the same is true of diabetes and sugar. Otherwise, allow your loved one to season food to his or her taste, as long as the doctor does not object.

One final issue that affects taste in dementia patients is oral hygiene. You may find that your loved one tries to dispose of his or her dentures at every opportunity. This may be because many people with dementia lose weight so that their dentures no longer fit comfortably. It may also be a negative reaction to having something that feels foreign placed in the mouth. Check several times a day to make sure that your loved one is still wearing his dentures. It is especially wise to check before you take the trash out, because many people with dementia simply wrap their dentures up in a napkin and throw them away. If your loved one is determined not to wear dentures, you may be able to reach a compromise. Ask him or her to wear dentures only while eating. At all other times, the dentures can remain safely in their storage container.

You also need to cue your loved one to brush his or her teeth after meals. Not only does this avoid the discomfort of cavities, it also helps clear away any bits of food that were not swallowed and minimizes any unpleasant aftertaste.

As you can see, if your loved one has dementia, paying attention to the five senses and how they are affected can be complicated. An optimal strategy is to involve a home care agency to give yourself a break. You may also want to contact an agency like the Alzheimer's Association (see Resources) to learn more about your loved one's condition and how to handle sensory loss and resultant behaviors.

CHAPTER 7: GRIEF, MOURNING, AND SENSORY LOSS

If your loved one has experienced sensory loss due to an illness, an accident, or as a part of the aging process, he or she is probably undergoing grieving and/or mourning.

What is the difference between grieving and mourning? According to Dr. Alan Wolfelt, who is the director at the Center for Life and Loss Transition, grieving is an internal process. It is defined by the feelings of sadness, numbness, loneliness, and despair that accompany a loss. Mourning is the outward expression of grieving. It includes behaviors like crying or wearing special clothes to signify that you have suffered a loss. Unfortunately, we live in a culture that has little tolerance for grieving and even less for mourning.

We want people to "snap out of it" or to "move on."

Maybe at some point you've even said something to your loved one like, "For goodness' sake, Mom, needing a hearing aid is not the end of the world" or "Don't worry about not being able to drive, Dad. We'll take you wherever you need to go."

If you have said words along those lines, don't be angry with yourself. Most caregivers make those types of remarks—with good intentions—at one time of another. This chapter will discuss helpful ways to respond to your loved one's sense of loss. It will also give you some markers to tell when grief has crossed the line into clinical depression, which requires an expert's help.

Primary Loss

There are two kinds of loss. The first is primary loss. Primary loss is easy for most people to understand. In involves losing something specific like your job, your spouse, or your eyesight. It's easy to be comforting and understanding, at least for a while, when someone suffers a primary loss.

Secondary Loss

Secondary losses, sometimes called symbolic losses, are pieces of yourself that slip away when a primary loss occurs. For instance, if your wife dies (primary loss), you lose the role of being a husband (secondary loss). Although they often go unacknowledged, the secondary losses surrounding sensory deficits can be significant.

A person losing her hearing may also have to face the fact that she is losing her youth. An avid reader, whose eyesight is failing due to macular degeneration, will suffer the secondary loss of no longer being able to enjoy his favorite activity.

Although secondary losses can be just as painful as primary losses, they tend to be misunderstood. Even the person who is grieving may downplay the importance of secondary losses.

You can support your loved one and help him or her recognize and grieve/mourn his or her symbolic losses by asking different variations of a single question: "How will that change your life?" You may have to ask this question more than once to get to the real source of grief. Here's an example of how such a conversation might play out:

Father: The doctor says he can't do any more to keep me from losing my eyesight.

You: Oh, Dad, I'm so sorry. That will mean some big changes in your life, won't it?

Father: Well, I won't be able to live alone anymore.

You: Probably not. We don't have to decide anything right now, but there are a lot of options open to you. You know you can always come live with us. How would you feel about that change?

Father (crying): I never wanted to be a burden on my children!

This is the secondary loss, the transition from being a self-sufficient, supportive parent to a "burden." Once the loss is out in the open, you can encourage your loved one to further express his feelings. Listen empathetically and try to understand how your father might feel, even if you don't see him as a burden in any way.

When you do speak, be sure to acknowledge all he has just said. "Dad, I hear that you don't want to become a burden. I love you and you would never be a burden to me, but if the idea of moving in with me upsets you so much, perhaps we can find other options that will keep you safe and independent."

Grief vs. Depression

The person who is grieving and the person who is depressed have several symptoms in common. They both feel sad or "blue" most of the time. Their sleeping and eating patterns may change. They may lose interest in activities they used to enjoy.

So how can you tell when healthy grieving and mourning cross the line into clinical depression? Even the experts don't always agree on the answer. According to the Diagnostic and Statistical Manual IV, a mental health professional can diagnose depression if grief has remained at the same level of intensity for more than two months. Some professionals, however, feel that two months is not nearly long enough to heal from a significant loss and will wait six months to a year before using the label, depression.

Almost anyone in the mental health field will immediately diagnose depression if your loved one starts talking about or planning to commit suicide.

Depression Statistics

In both Canada and the United States, depression statistics among senior citizens are grim. Both countries estimate that they are home to over 6 million people with late life depression. Of those people, only about 10% ever get the mental health help they need, in spite of the fact that depression is a highly treatable disease. In both countries, men over 65 represent the group most likely to die from suicide.

Suicide Warning Signs

Older people, who are experiencing sensory loss, may slip into a mindset of, "It can only get worse from here." They imagine themselves becoming more impaired, requiring more help, perhaps even winding up in a nursing facility because they need more can than their family can handle. For some of those people, suicide begins to look like a better option than continuing to live.

There is absolutely no way to be 100% sure who will attempt suicide and who will not—even the experts can't always tell.

Some people talk about suicide for years and never make an attempt; others kill themselves with little or no warning.

There are some signs that mental health professionals look for that indicate a high risk that a suicide attempt may occur. These include:

- Talking about suicide (about 70% of people who die by suicide have talked about killing themselves)
- Preoccupation with dying and death
- Obtaining the means to commit suicide such as buying a gun or hoarding pills
- Unable or unwilling to see or discuss any events in the future (may even say something like, "Oh, I don't think I'll be there to see that happen.")
- Expressing feelings of guilt or shame
- Getting affairs in order by making out a will, buying a burial plan, or giving away favorite possessions
- Saying goodbye to family and friends
- Withdrawing from social interaction
- Engaging in reckless behavior like driving too fast or mixing sleeping pills with alcohol
- Showing a sudden improvement in mood after being very down (because the decision has been reached and the person believes his or her pain will soon be over)

If you notice any of these warning signs, talk to your loved one in a calm, non-judgmental way. Ask your loved one directly if he or she is thinking about suicide. Don't be afraid to use the word suicide. You won't put any ideas in your loved one's head. In fact, he or she will probably be grateful you brought up the topic.

Listen to what your loved one has to say. Don't offer easy fixes or platitudes ("God never gives us more than we can handle") and don't make threats ("Keep talking like that and I'll put you in the mental hospital" or "If you commit suicide, you'll go to hell").

Just listen.

Sometimes, all your loved one needs is an opportunity to discharge all those feelings of grief, loss, and fear. Just being able to share some of the burden may bring enough relief to prevent suicide.

Assist your loved one with getting mental health help from a doctor, psychiatrist, psychotherapist, counselor, or member of the clergy. If your loved one remains suicidal or attempts to harm him or herself in front of you, call an ambulance and ask that she or he be transported to a psychiatric emergency room where he or she can receive much-needed care.

Treating Depression

Late life depression responds well to many different forms of treatment.

Older people can become depressed because they are lonely. Many of their friends have moved away or died, and they don't want to burden family with their problems. Sometimes the best intervention is to help your loved one get involved with a senior citizens' group like the Red Hat Society or volunteering. If nothing else, your loved one may enjoy spending part of the day at an adult daycare or senior health center.

If you can get your loved one up and moving, exercise is a wonderful antidepressant. Perhaps the two of you could take a walk every morning or join a community center to take a water aerobics class. Interacting with other seniors in the class may also help alleviate loneliness.

Psychotherapy, especially cognitive behavioral therapy (CBT) has a great track record for treating depression, but in order for the therapy to work, your loved one must be cognitively intact and able to remember advice and interventions from one session to the next. People with mid- to late-stage dementia are generally not good candidates for talk therapy.

Another option is medication, which can be prescribed by a general practitioner or psychiatrist. Make sure the person, who prescribes your loved one's medication, is aware of all of the other medications they take, even over the counter medications or herbal treatments. The doctor will probably start your loved one on a very low dose and slowly raise the amount until depression symptoms go away. Keep in mind that it may take three to four weeks to get the full benefit of an anti-depressant. Also, the first medication your loved one's doctor tries may not be effective. Sometimes, it takes two or three tries to find the antidepressant that works the best.

A final treatment, used as a last resort, is ECT or electroconvulsive therapy. You might have heard of it as electroshock therapy. Most people remember ECT as it was practiced in the 1950s. Back then, ECT was used as a method of social control. A much larger amount of electricity was passed through the brain, and the patient remained conscious throughout.

Today, patients are anesthetized and given a muscle relaxant before treatment. An electrode is used on only one side of the head, to lessen memory loss, and a very small amount of electrical current, just enough to induce a short seizure, is passed through your loved one's brain. After treatment, your loved one may suffer some confusion and memory loss, but these symptoms typically fade. To get the full benefit of the therapy, your loved one will have to undergo a number of treatments over a few weeks.

ECT is usually used when your loved one is profoundly depressed or suicidal and when other methods of therapy have failed.

Most people, especially if they have friends and family members to support them, grieve and mourn for the sensory losses they experience but are able to move on with their lives. Some people, however, may slip into depression and require professional treatment to deal with the sensory deficits they are experiencing.

CONCLUSION

As you can see, the processes that make it possible for the brain to receive information about what we're hearing, seeing, touching, smelling, or tasting are very complicated. If anything goes wrong with either the structure or function of the sensory organs, the result is sensory loss or distortion.

Not every senior citizen is affected by sensory loss. Those, who are affected, often manage to maintain their independence with the help of assistive devices and visits from family, friends, or caregivers. Unfortunately, some seniors have profound sensory loss, or sensory loss combined with another disease like Alzheimer's, and require 24/7 care and supervision.

What Should I Do if I Think My Loved One Has Sensory Loss?

The most respectful and helpful approach you can take is to share your observations with your loved one kindly but directly. ("Mom, I never see you embroider anymore. Are your eyes giving you trouble?" or "Dad, I've been here three days and in all that time you've scarcely touched your food. Is there something wrong?")

Your loved one may be reluctant to admit sensory loss out of fear of losing her independence or because of pride. You can help by reminding your loved one that many seniors live happy, healthy, and independent lives in spite of sensory loss.

If your loved one does admit to sensory loss or distortion, urge her to see her doctor. Ask if you can sit in on part of the appointment so you can listen to the doctor's recommendations and help brainstorm ways to keep them safe, healthy, and content. Rather than simply coming in with a plan, allow your loved one to express what would help her most.

If your loved one is agreeable, you may want to hire a caregiver to come over a few times a week to prepare meals, run errands, perform tasks your loved one has trouble with, and socialize.

Bringing up the issue of sensory loss with your loved one is not easy. You may need to broach the subject gently several times before your loved one is ready to discuss it with you. Once the problem is out on the table, however, you may be surprised at how easy it is to come up with solutions that will satisfy both you and the person you are concerned about.

Cheat Sheet—Quick Tips for Talking about Sensory Loss with Your Loved One

- Approach your loved one at a time when you are both calm and can expect at least half an hour of privacy.
- State observations, not accusations (Rather than saying, "Aunt June, you stink," try, "Aunt June, I'm noticing a slight odor of urine in here. Is it bothering you, too?")
- Give your loved one time to share his or her point of view.
- Ask your loved one what he or she thinks might help.
- Make it clear that some issues are not negotiable. (Rather than saying, "Don't you think you should see the eye doctor?" try, "I'm going to make an appointment for you to see Dr. Jones. Do mornings or afternoons work best for you?")
- Walk away. If the conversation is going nowhere or you're just getting frustrated, walk away and approach the topic another day.

- Once the sensory loss has been acknowledged, check in with your loved one regularly to see how he or she is doing.
- Get help for yourself. Whether you live with your loved one or six states away, it's still stressful to be a caregiver. Finding a caregiver support group for yourself is a great start. So is bringing in another family member or hiring someone to help with your loved one's care.

If you're looking for a very special kind of caregiver, the next chapter explains why Home Care Assistance is the place to go when your loved one requires extra care.

Home Care Assistance: Balanced Care Method Makes the Difference

People are living longer and healthier lives today than they ever have in the past. It is not unusual for seniors to remain active and independent well into their 80s and 90s. Some older people, however, do develop health problems and severe sensory deficits that make it necessary for them to rely on another person for all or part of their care.

If that day comes for your loved one, we hope you will make our care managers at Home Care Assistance your partners in caregiving. Home Care Assistance is North America's leading provider of in-home care for seniors. Over the years, we've helped over 100,000 families navigate their care options. Whether your loved one is facing frailty, chronic illness, reduced mobility or memory loss, Home Care Assistance caregivers are here to help. With services customized to the unique needs of every client, we provide security and independence to seniors and peace of mind to their families.

Our caregivers are experienced professionals who are trained to provide one-on-one assistance that allows our clients to live happier, healthier lives at home. They come directly to the home and help with:

- Mobility
- Meal Preparation
- Transportation
- Medication Reminders
- Companionship
- Exercise
- Mental stimulation
- Bathing and Grooming
- Dressing
- Transferring
- and More

We work with you to establish a regular schedule so you know exactly who to expect, and when. Our caregivers are available when you need them, whether it's a few hours at a time or 24/7...and our care managers are on call day or night to answer questions and respond to issues. Home Care Assistance is unique in the senior care industry in that we:

- Hire only 1 in 25 applicants and conduct extensive screening and background checks
- Protect our clients by assuming liability for our caregivers as employees and not contractors
- Train our caregivers in our proprietary Balanced Care Method, a unique approach to senior care that promotes healthy mind, body and spirit
- Adhere to a rigorous client to care manager ratio that contributes to our 97% client satisfaction rate

- Serve as preferred providers for professionals in the medical and senior communities, including hospitals and Alzheimer's centers
- Maintain our long-standing reputation as recognized experts in senior care with a series of consumer education books, publications, webinars and guides

When you're ready to take the next step, our Care Manager will meet with you and assess your loved one's needs. We work together to select the perfect caregiver and develop a care plan that meets with everyone's approval. After services begin, our ongoing care management, quality assurance visits and status reporting ensure that our clients are 100% satisfied every step of the way. Home Care Assistance offers you a stress free solution that doesn't force you to choose between becoming a caregiver yourself and placing your loved one in a facility.

The Balanced Care Method™

All Home Care Assistance caregivers are trained using the company's unique Balanced Care Method ™, a home care approach that emphasizes moderation and variety. Just as we discussed in Section 5 (Taste), our caregivers learn how important it is for seniors to have good nutrition. They introduce a diet that is flavorful, rich in different textures, and full of vitamins, fiber, proteins, and omega-3 fatty acids. They also help clients engage in stretching their muscles or low-impact exercise to keep them physically independent as long as possible.

Other hallmarks of the Balanced Care Method™ include:
- Meeting a client's social needs though conversations, outings, and assistance staying in touch with friends and family members

- Providing all personal care in a sensitive way that allows clients to maintain their privacy and dignity
- Providing food, activities, and interactions that appeal to all of the senses

If you would like to contact Home Care Assistance to see if there is an agency in your area or to discuss your loved one's care, you can reach us through our website at **http://www.homecareassistance.com** or via email at **info@homecareassistance.com**. You can also send a letter to our corporate headquarters: Home Care Assistance, 148 Hawthorne Avenue, Palo Alto, CA 94301.

APPENDIX A:
HEALTHCARE AND REHABILITATION PROFESSIONALS

Audiologist – health professional trained in diagnosing and treating problems with balance and hearing; an audiologist helps seniors select appropriate hearing aids.

Counselor – a mental health professional who evaluates, supports, and instructs individuals with emotional or developmental concerns; usually consulted to help overcome a single problem or issue.

Dentist – a medical professional who diagnoses and treats problems with the teeth, gums, and the underlying bone.

Dietitian – a health professional who promotes good health through proper diet and who advocates the therapeutic use of diet to treat disease.

ENT – see otolaryngologist.

Family doctor – see general practitioner.

General practitioner – a physician with no declared specialty, who treats a variety of medical problems in people of all ages.

Gerontologist – a healthcare provider trained in assessing and meeting the needs of senior clients.

Caregiver – a worker specifically trained and certified to provide non-medical personal (physical) care under the supervision of a registered nurse.

Homemaker – a worker, who assists with tasks like light-housekeeping, meal preparation, laundry services, and monitoring conditions in the home but does not provide personal (physical) care.

Licensed practical nurse (LPN) – a nurse, who has completed a practical nursing program and is state-licensed to provide routine care to patients under the direction of a registered nurse or a physician.

Neurologist – a doctor, who specializes in disorders of the brain and central nervous system.

Neurosurgeon – a surgeon, who specializes in managing diseases and injuries involving the brain, the spinal cord, and the peripheral nerves.

Occupational therapist – an allied health professional, who provides assessment and treatment directed towards helping clients develop skills of daily living; also works on the development of sensory motor perception and skills.

Ophthalmologist – a physician, usually a surgeon, who specializes in diagnosing and treating defects, injuries, and disorders of the eye; your loved one might see this type of eye specialist for cataract removal.

Optician – A professional, who designs and makes optical instruments or lenses such as eyeglasses.

Optometrist – a medical professional, who examines and tests the eyes for disease and who treats refractive disorders by prescribing corrective lenses.

Oral and maxillofacial surgeon – a dentist, who specializes in surgical reconstruction of facial deformities caused by disease or trauma.

Orthotist – a health care professional, who is skilled in making and fitting orthopedic appliances.

Otolaryngologist – a doctor, who specializes in the diagnosis and treatment of diseases involving the ears, nose, and throat.

Physical therapist – an allied health professional, who uses exercise, application of heat and cold, and other physical treatments to increase independence and mobility.

Podiatrist – a health professional, who diagnoses and treats problems with the feet; also provides routine foot care to diabetics and others who are at an increased risk of infection of the lower extremities.

Prosthetist – a person who creates and fits artificial limbs and similar devices.

Prosthodontist – a dentist, who specializes in restoring and replacing teeth with devices such as crowns, caps, bridges, veneers, dentures, and implants.

Psychiatrist – a physician, who specializes in diagnosing and treating mental health problems; seniors who are depressed, anxious, or showing signs of cognitive decline are often referred to psychiatrists.

Psychologist – a specialist in the study of the structure and function of the brain, who provides testing, assessment, and psychotherapy to people with mental, emotional or cognitive disorders; your loved one may see a psychologist for treatment of depression and anxiety.

Registered nurse (RN) – a graduate-trained nurse, who has passed a state exam and holds a license to practice nursing.

Rehabilitation nurse – Registered nurse, who cares for patients, who are experiencing temporary or permanent disabilities that are extensive enough to disrupt the patient's functioning and lifestyle.

Rhinologist – a physician, who specializes in the diagnosis and treatment of illnesses and disorders of the nose.

Social worker – a professional, who provides counseling, emotional support, and referrals to community resources to assist clients, who are experiencing medical or other psychosocial problems.

Speech therapist – a professional, who provides assessments and treats patients with disorders in speech, language, and swallowing.

APPENDIX B: HELPFUL BOOKS FOR SENIORS AND/OR CAREGIVERS

Alzheimer's and Related Dementias

The 36-Hour Day: A Family Guide to Caring for People Who Have Alzheimer Disease, Related Dementias, and Memory Loss (5th Edition), by Nancy L. Mace and Peter V. Rabins (The Johns Hopkins University Press, 2011).

A Caregiver's Guide to Alzheimer's Disease: 300 Tips for Making Life Easier, by Patricia Callone, Barbara Vasiloff, Roger Brumback, Janaan Manternach, and Connie Kudlacek (Demos Medical Publishing, 2005).

A Caregiver's Guide to Lewy Body Dementia, by Helen Buell Whitworth and Jim Whitworth (Demos Health, 2010).
A Dignified Life: The Best Friends Approach to Alzheimer's Care, A Guide for Family Caregivers, by Virginia Bell and David Troxel (HCI, 2002).

Keeping Busy: A Handbook of Activities for Persons with Dementia, by James R. Dowling (The Johns Hopkins University Press, 1995).

Loving Someone Who Has Dementia: How to Find Hope While Coping with Stress and Grief, by Pauline Boss (Jossey-Bass, 2011).

Talking to Alzheimer's: Simple Ways to Connect When You Visit with a Family Member or Friend, by Claudia J. Strauss (New Harbinger Publications, 2002).

Family Communication

How to Say It to Seniors: Closing the Communication Gap with Our Elders, by David Solie (Prentice Hall Press, 2004).

The Parent Care Conversation: Six Strategies for Dealing with the Emotional and Financial Challenges of Aging Parents, by Dan Taylor (Penguin, 2006).

Talking to Depression: Simple Ways to Connect When Someone in Your Life is Depressed, by Claudia J. Strauss (NAL Trade, 2004).

When Children Grieve: For Adults to Help Children Deal with Death, Divorce, Pet Loss, Moving, and Other Losses, by John W. James, Russell Friedman, and Leslie Matthews (Harper Perennial, 2002).

Help for the Caregiver

American Medical Association Guide to Home Caregiving, by the American Medical Association (Wiley, 2001).

The Complete Eldercare Planner, Revised and Updated Edition: Where to Start, Which Questions to Ask, and How to Find Help, by Joy Loverde (Three Rivers Press, 2009).

Elder Rage or Take My Father, Please!: How to Survive Caring for Aging Parents, by Jacqueline Marcell (Impressive Press, 2001).

Eldercare for Dummies, by Rachelle Zukerman (For Dummies, 2003).

The Emotional Survival Guide for Caregivers: Looking after Yourself and Your Family While Helping an Aging Parent, by Barry J. Jacobs (The Guilford Press, 2006).

From Hospital to Home Care: A Step by Step Guide to Providing Care to Patients Post Hospitalization, by Kathy N. Johnson, James H. Johnson, and Lily Sarafan (Home Care Press, 2012).

The Good Caregiver: A One-of-a-Kind Compassionate Resource for Anyone Caring for Aging Loved Ones, by Robert L. Kane (Avery Trade, 2011).

The Handbook of Live-in Care: A Guide for Caregivers, by Kathy N. Johnson, James H. Johnson, and Lily Sarafan (Home Care Press, 2011).

How You Can Survive When They're Depressed: Living and Coping with Depression Fallout, by Anne Sheffield (Three Rivers Press, 1999).

Making the Moments Count: Leisure Activities for Caregiving Relationships, by Joanne Ardolf Decker (The Johns Hopkins University Press, 1997).

Help for the Older Adult

How to Be Sick: A Buddhist-Inspired Guide for the Chronically Ill and Their Caregivers, by Toni Bernhard (Wisdom Publications, 2010).

Macular Disease: Practical Strategies for Living with Vision Loss, by Peggy R. Wolfe (Park Publishing, Inc., 2011).

The Mindful Way through Depression: Freeing Yourself from Chronic Unhappiness, by Mark Williams, John Teasdale, Zindel Segal, and Jon Kabat-Zinn (The Guilford Press, 2007).

The Mindfulness and Acceptance Workbook for Depression: Using Acceptance and Commitment Therapy to Move through Depression and Create a Life Worth Living, by Patricia J. Robinson and Kirk D. Strosahl (New Harbinger Publications, 2008).

Recovery from Losses in Life, by H. Norman Wright (Revell, 2006).

Simple Circles: An Exercise Program for Seniors and Their Families, by Howie Bell (CreateSpace, 2011).

Stronger after Stroke: Your Roadmap to Recovery, by Peter G. Levine (Demos Health, 2008).

APPENDIX C:
WEB-BASED RESOURCES FOR SENIORS
AND/OR CAREGIVERS

AARP - http://www.aarp.org
Provides political advocacy, discounts, and information to senior citizens

Agency for Healthcare Research and Quality -
http://www.ahrq.gov/research/elderix.htm
Reviews the results of evidence-based healthcare studies about seniors

Alzheimer's Association - http://www.alz.org
Funds research and provides information and support to families dealing with Alzheimer's

Canadian Caregiver Coalition - http://www.ccc-ccan.ca
Provides advocacy, leadership, research, education, information, communication and resource development to caregivers in Canada

Canadian Dementia Action Network - http://www.cdan.ca
Dedicated to finding a cure as well, as helping those currently living with dementia and their families

Home Care Assistance - http://www.homecareassistance.com
Provides non-medical in-home care to seniors

Hospital to Home Care – http://hospitaltohomecare.com
Provides information on post-hospitalization care

Medicare.gov - http://www.medicare.gov
Provides information about government-backed health programs

Seniors Canada Online - http://www.seniors.gc.ca
Information and services for Canadian seniors

National Family Caregivers Association -
http://www.nfcacares.org
Offering education, support, empowerment and advocacy to
caregivers

National Institute on Aging - http://www.nia.nih.gov
Conducts geriatric research and provides information to seniors
and their families

Public Health Agency of Canada, Aging and Seniors -
http://www.phac-aspc.gc.ca/seniors-aines
Provides medical information for Canadian Seniors

USA.gov., Senior Citizens' Resources -
http://www.usa.gov/Topics/Seniors
List of links to other resources dealing with health care, caregiver
resources, and end of life issues

OUR MISSION

Our mission at Home Care Assistance is to change the way the world ages. We provide older adults with quality care that enables them to live happier, healthier lives at home. Our services are distinguished by the caliber of our caregivers, the responsiveness of our staff and our expertise in Live-In care. We embrace a positive, balanced approach to aging centered on the evolving needs of older adults.

- Live-In Experts. We specialize in around the clock care to help seniors live well at home.

- Available 24/7. Care managers are on call for clients and their families, even during nights and weekends.

- High Caliber Caregivers. We hire only 1 in 25 applicants and provide ongoing training and supervision.

- Balanced Care. Our unique approach to care promotes healthy mind, body and spirit.

- No Long Term Contracts. Use our services only as long as you're 100% satisfied.

- A Trusted Partner. We're honored to be Preferred Providers for professionals in both the medical and senior communities.

- Peace of Mind. Independent industry surveys place our client satisfaction rate at 97%.

AUTHOR BIOGRAPHIES

Kathy N. Johnson, PhD, CMC is a Certified Geriatric Care Manager and Chief Executive Officer of Home Care Assistance. A recognized leader in senior care, she holds a Doctorate in Psychology from the Illinois Institute of Technology.

James H. Johnson, PhD is a licensed clinical psychologist and Chairman of Home Care Assistance. He is the former department chair of the Virginia Consortium for Professional Psychology and the award-winning author of nine books. He holds a Doctorate in Psychology from the University of Minnesota.

Lily Sarafan, MS is President and Chief Operating Officer of Home Care Assistance. She has been featured as an industry expert by more than 100 media outlets. She holds Masters and Bachelors degrees from Stanford University.

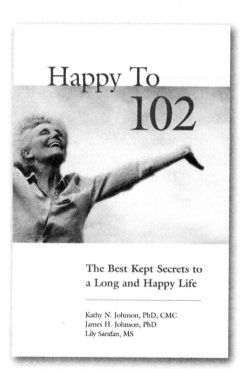

Available on **amazon**.com.

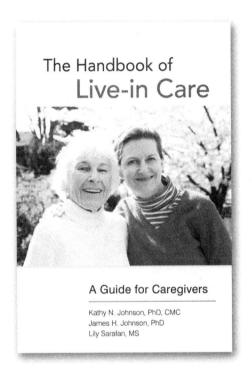

Available on amazon.com®

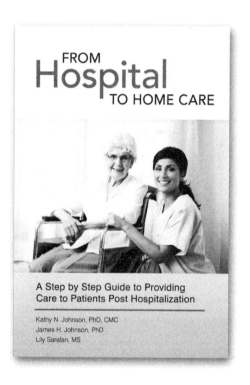

Available on **amazon**.com.

NOTES

NOTES

NOTES

NOTES

NOTES

NOTES

NOTES

NOTES

NOTES

NOTES

NOTES